The Complete Guide to Taming Chronic Inflammation

The Complete Guide to Taming Chronic Inflammation

An 8-step Action Plan to Naturally Ease Inflammation, Harmonize Your Immune System, Nurture Gut Health, Manage Stress, and Achieve Daily Well-being

Written by: Tara Miles

www.SmartMindPublishing.com

First edition, 2024
    ISBN 978-1-916662-22-3 (paperback)
    ISBN 978-1-916662-23-0 (ebook)
    ISBN 978-1-916662-24-7 (hardback)

Publisher's Bookstore: www.smartmindpublishing.com
Email: tara.miles.author@gmail.com

Table of content

Ready to take your wellbeing journey to the next level?

This Journal is Here for You.

The 30-Day Guided Workbook Journal is your perfect companion for staying on track and building lasting, beneficial habits.

Designed to complement the strategies in this book, the journal offers practical tools to help you **monitor daily progress**, reflect on your journey, and make adjustments where needed. With dedicated space to **track new habits, log improvements, and keep yourself accountable**, this workbook ensures you stay motivated and focused on achieving your well-being goals.

Use it as a powerful resource to support your transformation to a healthier, inflammation-free life.

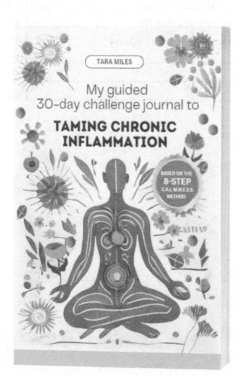

Just scan this QR code with your phone to land directly on the journal's Amazon page,

or visit the Publisher's bookstore at www.smartmindpublishing.com

Introduction

As the alarm blares to signal the start of another day, you reach out to silence it only to be greeted by the familiar ache in your joints. Barely out of bed, the soreness reminds you that today, like so many others, will be filled with chronic aches, fatigue, and the struggle to accomplish even the simplest tasks. Sound familiar? If so, you're not alone. In fact, three out of five people worldwide are right there with you, fighting the relentless frustrations of chronic inflammation. And here's a staggering fact: a whopping 80% of all major human diseases are fueled by inflammation.

Let's talk about the toll it takes – physically, emotionally, and mentally. It's not just about the pain, it's about how it infiltrates every aspect of your life. It can put strain on your relationships, dampen work performance, and rob you of the joy in everyday activities. I get it, it's tough. And to make matters worse, the sea of conflicting health advice out there can leave you feeling utterly lost and alone.

But first, take a deep breath. Deep breath... We're in this together, and if you've found your way here that means you're ready for a change. You're ready to say enough is enough and take back control of your health. Whether it's a nagging pain or a simple desire for a better quality of life that brought you here, the journey to healing starts with understanding what's going on inside your body. Rest assured, I will guide you along the way.

So, what exactly is inflammation? Think of it as your body's way of raising a red flag when something's not quite right – whether it's an injury, illness, or an unwelcome guest like toxins or germs. Understanding inflammation is the first step toward finding relief from the constant discomfort and stress it brings along.

Enter the eight-step C.A.L.M.N.E.S.S. framework – your trusty guide on this journey to reclaiming your vitality and well-being. Each step serves as a bright beacon of hope, shining light on practical strategies to battle your inflammation head-on. From understanding the ins and outs of inflammation to crafting your personalized action plan, consider this your roadmap to a life free from the frustration and struggles of chronic pain.

C.A.L.M.N.E.S.S Steps

- **C: Comprehend Inflammation** - Let's dive deep into the world of inflammation together so we can learn what causes it, how it shows up in your body, and what triggers it. Armed with this knowledge, we can start unraveling the mystery behind your pain and find ways to ease it.

- **A: Adjust Your Diet** - Food is medicine. And with that in mind, we'll explore the power of anti-inflammatory foods as well as how to weave them into your diet while giving those inflammatory culprits a gentle nudge out the door. Who knew eating your way to better health could be so delicious?

- **L: Leverage Movement** - Movement isn't just about hitting the gym; it's about finding joy in motion. Let's discover fun ways to get your body moving, whether it's dancing in your living room or taking a leisurely stroll in the park. Exercise doesn't have to be a chore; it can be a celebration of what your body can do.

- **M: Manage Stress** - Stress is inflammation's sneaky sidekick, always lurking in the shadows. Together, we'll uncover simple yet effective stress-busting techniques, from deep breathing exercises to finding moments of calm in the chaos of everyday life. Because when you're at peace, inflammation doesn't stand a chance.

- **N: Nurture Sleep** - Ah, the sweet embrace of sleep. Let's make sure you're getting the quality shut-eye your body craves, with bedtime rituals and cozy sleep environments that set the stage for restorative rest. Because when you wake up feeling refreshed, you're ready to take on the day – inflammation and all.

- **E: Enhance Lifestyle Choices** - It's time to make choices that support your well-being by ditching unhealthy habits to embrace activities that bring you joy. Small changes can add up to big results, and we're here to cheer you on every step of the way.

- **S: Seek Natural Remedies** - Mother Nature often knows best. We'll explore the world of natural remedies, from herbal supplements to holistic therapies, to find what works best for you. Because when it comes to healing, sometimes the simplest solutions are the most effective.

- **S: Solidify Your Action Plan** - Armed with all of this newfound knowledge, it's time to craft your personalized action plan – the roadmap to living a life free from chronic inflammation. Together, we'll outline the steps you need to take to reclaim your health and well-being, one day at a time.

So, are you ready to embark on this journey toward a brighter, pain-free tomorrow together? We've laid out a framework in this book that will give you a deeper understanding of inflammation and how to create a path of healing personalized just for you! Each step brings you closer to a life free from discomfort and filled with vitality. You'll gain insights into identifying your triggers, discovering anti-inflammatory foods, and unlocking the shortcuts that will work for you and revolutionize your health and lifestyle.

It won't be easy, but I promise you won't be alone. Together, we'll navigate the ups and downs, celebrate the victories, and find joy in the journey. Because, when it comes to healing, having a support system and a guide to help you, is just like having a friend by your side. Together we will begin this healing journey toward a pain-free life. Welcome to your transformational journey – let's get started.

Chapter 1 - C.A.L.M.N.E.S.S.

C - Comprehend Inflammation and Know Your Friend (or Enemy)

In a perfect world, every day wouldn't feel like being a contestant on "Survivor: Chronic Inflammation Edition," where each morning brings new challenges, from dodging germs like a pro to outsmarting pain triggers like a seasoned contestant. But we're not just battling for the immunity statue, are we? We're searching for vitality, pain-free days, and a sense of overall well-being. We all feel the struggle as we battle through the day, trying to ward off viruses and bacteria. When you're dealing with inflammation, the battle feels never-ending and overwhelming, and it can seem like a constant fight to survive. Life shouldn't be this way, but you're not alone in feeling like you're in survival mode every day.

Together, we can untangle the mysteries of inflammation and arm ourselves with the knowledge needed to live a life that gets us out of 'survival mode'. Understanding inflammation will help us defeat this battle we call life, so we can feel more at ease, more like ourselves, and truly enjoy each day to the fullest. Let us dive in and learn about inflammation – what it is, where it comes from, and, ultimately, how it can affect us if we don't take charge.

What is Inflammation?

Inflammation is like your body's own superhero response team, jumping into action whenever it senses trouble. In scientific terms, it's a complex biological process that helps your body fight off invaders like bacteria, viruses, and other harmful substances. Picture it as a team of microscopic firefighters rushing to the scene of a blaze, ready to extinguish the flames and restore order. But what's interesting is that inflammation isn't just about battling external threats; it also plays a crucial role in healing injuries and repairing damaged tissues. These microscopic response teams known as white blood cells are on call whenever anything foreign enters your body whether that be through bacteria, an open wound, or some other underlying result of damage in or to your body, these white blood cells are our immune system's top line of defense.

Imagine inflammation as your body's way of saying, "Hey, something's off and doesn't feel quite right here, but I'm gonna do whatever it takes to fix it!" It's like your internal alarm system, warning you of potential dangers and mobilizing the troops to keep you safe. But there's a catch: sometimes, this response can get a little overenthusiastic and they begin to see danger around every corner. This means your white blood cells, or these microscopic superheroes, double down and go into the process of overprotecting every part of your body, including parts that don't need protection. And this is when inflammation can become chronic, causing more harm than good and leaving you feeling like you're stuck in a never-ending battle.

Understanding the difference between acute and chronic inflammation is the first step toward regaining control. Acute inflammation is short-lived; it kicks in quickly, does its job, and then backs off once the threat is neutralized. It's your body's way of handling immediate dangers, like a swift ninja that takes out the bad guys before they can do any damage. Chronic inflammation, on the other hand, is like a relentless siege, it lingers long after the initial threat has passed, wreaking havoc on your body and leaving you feeling drained and defeated.

Let's delve deeper into the world of inflammation, and remember this: it's not just about fighting off invaders; it's about finding the balance between protection and overreaction. By arming ourselves with knowledge and understanding, we can turn the tide in our favor, reclaim our health and vitality, and ultimately get out of "survival mode."

Acute vs. Chronic Inflammation

Acute Inflammation

As mentioned, acute inflammation is a short-term response to an injury or virus. It's like when you scrape your knee on the pavement after tripping over the yellow line in the road – we've all been there. Regardless of how it happens, the skin is torn, becoming red and sensitive to the touch, and it might even burn or sting. Within a few hours, it scabs over and begins to bruise, all the while causing pain along the inflamed skin and tissue. This is acute inflammation in action. But don't worry, because it's temporary; it will heal and stop hurting in due time.

Acute inflammation is your body's way of swiftly responding to a threat, like a first responder leaping into action at the first sign of trouble. It's a rapid and efficient process that helps to clear away any debris, repair damaged tissues, and restore your body to its former glory. So, the next time you find yourself nursing a scraped knee or a pesky bug bite, remember – acute inflammation is just your body's way of showing that it's hard at work, your white blood cells are fighting off the invaders and getting you back on your feet.

If needed, you can help your defense system and reduce your discomfort by taking an over-the-counter pain reliever or using a cold compress alongside herbal remedies to alleviate pain and swelling.

In the case of a bacterial infection, antibiotics often help win the battle. These are helpful when your immune system has already been weakened or is being overwhelmed by a foreign agent, such as an infection. While your body is taking action, sometimes it's just not enough for that particular battle, and intervention is necessary. When the battle is intense, our bodies can get overloaded, leading us to worse chronic inflammation and contributing to the onset of many other illnesses and diseases.

Understand what has caused your acute inflammation, a wound, injury, infection, and so forth, and then treat it the best you can right away, regardless of whether that means rest, herbal treatments, home remedies, medication, or a combination of several treatments. Otherwise, it can transform into a vicious circle of inflammation and chronic conditions.

Chronic Inflammation

Chronic inflammation is like that friend who just can't take a hint – it sticks around way longer than it should, causing more trouble than it solves. Your body's defense system, always eager to jump into action, revs up the production of white blood cells and chemical messengers to tackle injuries or illnesses. But sometimes, it can get a little too enthusiastic and instead decide to keep the party going, leading to chronic inflammation. It's like having an overzealous security guard who sees danger lurking in every corner, even where there's none to be found. As a result, your body remains in a perpetual state of alert, with its defenders turning into unwitting villains, attacking healthy tissue and organs in the process.

Unlike acute inflammation, which responds fast, does what it needs too, and then leaves on cue, chronic inflammation is the unwelcome guest that overstays its welcome. It's stealthy, often invisible, and sneaky, there's no obvious culprit to blame. But of course, there's always a cause or a combination of causes lurking beneath the surface. Throughout this book, we'll embark on a mission to identify and neutralize these troublemakers, while also preventing new ones from wreaking havoc down the line. Sometimes, it's our own lifestyle choices or unavoidable circumstances, like our jobs, that unwittingly feed the flames of chronic inflammation. For example, long-term exposure to chemicals, toxins, or secondhand smoke can wreak havoc on our DNA and fatty tissues, fast-tracking us to the golden years of aging and, of course, feeding inflammation.

Our bodies are pretty smart, they know when something's wrong and aren't shy about sounding the alarm. Inflammation can be triggered by a variety of activities and exposures, from smoking and alcohol to stress and sleepless nights. It's our body's way of saying, "Hey, something's wrong!" But here's the kicker: chronic inflammation isn't just a nuisance; it's a sign that something deeper is going on, something that demands our attention before it snowballs into something worse. The sad truth is that inflammation-related diseases can account for a whopping 50% of all global deaths, ranging from cardiovascular disease to Alzheimer's and everything in between. Can you believe it? So getting your inflammation under control now is key to preventing worse issues including early death.

Here are just some of the diseases fueled by chronic inflammation:

- Cardiovascular disease
- Stroke
- Cancer
- Diabetes
- Rheumatoid arthritis
- Chron's
- Chronic kidney disease
- Asthma and allergies
- Alzheimer's
- Metabolic syndrome
- Multiple autoimmune syndrome

So, inflammation isn't the disease itself; rather it's more like a sidekick, sometimes helpful, periodically causing more trouble than it's worth. It's a warning sign alerting us to underlying issues that need addressing right away. So, what's a person to do when faced with constant pain and discomfort? One thing we can do is roll up our sleeves and get some testing done. Tests like the C-reactive protein (CRP) blood test can clue us in on inflammation levels, while the erythrocyte sedimentation rate (ESR) test can help identify conditions like rheumatoid arthritis. But remember, no matter what the test results say, if you're stuck in a cycle of chronic pain, chances are, chronic inflammation is the offender. And, you can take hold now by understanding what kind of inflammation you have, arming yourself with the right tools so you can stop inflammation in its tracks.

Here are some signs of chronic inflammation:

- Balance issues
- Insulin resistance
- Muscle aches
- Diarrhea
- Chronic lower back pain
- Feeling tired all the time
- Hardening of the arteries
- Blood clotting
- Dry eye
- Brain issues
- Livedo Reticularis

From acute to chronic inflammation. Your body's mixed signals

Our bodies are smart and almost always know what to do, but that doesn't mean that we can't get mixed signals that cause confusion and overreaction from our immune system. You see, chronic inflammation often starts off as the body's valiant attempt to fend off dangerous intruders like viruses, bacteria, or injury which as discussed is called acute inflammation. But here's the catch: if the immune system doesn't get the memo to stand down once the threat is vanquished, that's when inflammation can spiral out of control and chronic inflammation begins to settle in. This means when you should be healed and good to go the workers keep on going fighting to the point of damaging things.

Imagine this: acute inflammation, our body's trusty sidekick, swoops in to save the day, battling viruses, bacteria, and other nasties like a hero in an action movie. But if it overstays its welcome, it morphs into chronic inflammation before you know it, becoming more of a problem than a savior. It's like the body's immune system is stuck on repeat, unable to turn itself off. And just like that, acute inflammation has now transitioned into chronic inflammation.

Now, let's talk about the consequences of this prolonged inflammation party. Chronic inflammation isn't just a one-trick pony; it's rather a master of disguise, infiltrating various systems and wreaking havoc wherever it goes, from cancer to heart disease, type 2 diabetes to cognitive decline and dementia in older adults. Of course, genetics, age, weight, hormones, and stress can also play a major role but only as a contributing factor. Nonetheless, it can be accelerated by untreated or mistreated acute symptoms. In addition, we can activate inflammatory responses from triggers like bad habits and environments, as well as possible food sensitivities; all of which can feed inflammation. Chronic inflammation doesn't discriminate – it's the ultimate equal-opportunity troublemaker; it does where it wants, takes what it needs, and expands to wherever it wants.

The good news is that with a better understanding of inflammation, you can now arm yourself with an arsenal of tools, from lifestyle changes to cutting-edge treatments, to help you kick chronic inflammation to the curb and usher in a new era of vitality and well-being. Your body is saying something is wrong, and you need to take action;

Throughout the rest of the book, we will talk directly about the real changes you can make every day to amp up your fight toward pain-free days and nights. Now you know that inflammation is a symptom and a mechanism to deal with something deeper and you can take action to arm yourself and take action to ease your pain.

Each chapter will include a checklist to guide you through the main takeaways, encouraging reflection on any personal health symptoms or experiences that might indicate chronic inflammation.

How to Use the Chapter Checklists?

This chapter checklist is designed to help you review and apply the key concepts covered in the chapter. Here's how to make the most of it:

1. Reflect on Key Points: Take a moment to go through each item on the checklist. Reflect on what you've learned and how it applies to your own situation. Consider any new insights or strategies you might have gained.

2. Assess Your Situation: For each checklist item, think about how it relates to your health and well-being. Are there areas where you could improve or apply new techniques? Use this as an opportunity to evaluate your current habits and identify areas for growth.

3. Take Notes: Jot down any thoughts, observations, or actionable steps that come to mind as you work through the checklist. This can help you create a personalized plan based on the chapter's content.

4. Set Goals: Based on your notes, set specific, actionable goals to address any areas where you want to make changes. This could include trying new stress management techniques, adjusting your sleep habits, or incorporating different self-care practices.

5. Review Regularly: Revisit the checklist periodically to track your progress and make adjustments as needed. Regular review can help you stay on track and continue to make improvements over time.

By using this checklist, you'll be better equipped to apply what you've learned and take meaningful steps toward enhancing your well-being.

Understanding Inflammation Checklist

Understand the basic role of inflammation in the body:

- ☐ Learn about inflammation's role as the body's natural defense mechanism.
- ☐ Explore how inflammation helps to fight off infections and heal injuries.
- ☐ Gain insight into the importance of inflammation for overall health and well-being.

Distinguish between acute and chronic inflammation:

- ☐ Differentiate between acute inflammation, a short-term response to injury or infection, and chronic inflammation, a prolonged and often harmful state.
- ☐ Identify the key differences in how acute and chronic inflammation manifest in the body.
- ☐ Understand the transition from acute to chronic inflammation and its implications for long-term health.

Recognize the signs that might indicate chronic inflammation:

- ☐ Learn to identify common signs and symptoms of chronic inflammation, such as persistent pain, fatigue, and digestive issues.
- ☐ Understand how chronic inflammation can contribute to the development of various health conditions, including cardiovascular disease, diabetes, and autoimmune disorders.
- ☐ Reflect on personal experiences and health concerns to assess whether chronic inflammation may be a contributing factor to overall health challenges.

Self-Assessment Inflammation Questionnaire

Take a moment to assess your current health status with our inflammation questionnaire. This interactive tool will guide you through a series of questions designed to help you evaluate potential signs of inflammation in your body.

Please answer the following questions honestly and to the best of your ability.

1. General Health

- How would you rate your overall health on a scale of 1 to 10, with 1 being poor and 10 being excellent?
- Do you often experience fatigue or lack of energy?
- Have you noticed any changes in your appetite or weight recently?

2. Pain and Discomfort

- Do you experience frequent pain in your joints or muscles?
- Are you prone to headaches or migraines?
- Do you have digestive issues, such as bloating, gas, or abdominal pain?

3. Physical Symptoms

- Have you noticed any changes in your skin, such as redness, itching, or rashes?
- Do you experience frequent colds, infections, or allergies?
- Have you been diagnosed with any chronic health conditions, such as arthritis or diabetes?

4. Lifestyle Factors

- Do you consume tobacco products?
- How would you rate your stress levels on a scale of 1 to 10, with 1 being low and 10 being high?
- Do you engage in regular physical activity or exercise?

5. Diet and Nutrition

- How would you describe your typical diet? (e.g., high in processed foods, balanced with fruits and vegetables)
- Do you consume sugary or high-fat foods regularly?
- Are you able to maintain a healthy weight?

6. Sleep Quality

- Do you have trouble falling asleep or staying asleep?
- How many hours of sleep do you typically get each night?
- Do you wake up feeling rested and refreshed?

7. Medical History

- Have you been diagnosed with any inflammatory conditions, such as rheumatoid arthritis or Crohn's disease?
- Are you currently taking any medications or supplements for inflammation or related symptoms?
- Have you undergone any recent medical tests or procedures related to inflammation?

Once you've completed the questionnaire, take some time to review your responses and consider any patterns or trends that may indicate inflammation. Remember, this questionnaire is not a diagnostic tool but a helpful starting point for evaluating your health. If you have concerns about inflammation or related symptoms, we recommend consulting with a healthcare professional for personalized guidance and treatment options.

Chapter 2 - C.**A**.L.M.N.E.S.S.

A - Adjust Your Diet & Eat Your Way to Calm

It can be disheartening in a world full of disinformation and false claims, a gimmick around every corner. However, the more we connect with people who are also suffering, we will find inspiring stories to uplift and encourage us on our journey toward healing. One of many inspiring stories comes from Janice, a participant in my Healthy Habits Workshop. She not only lost over 20 pounds but has also overcome a lifetime of skin inflammation, an acute disorder that had become chronic.

As a teenager, Janice battled minor skin irritations and seasonal eczema flare-ups that made her dread stepping outside. The embarrassment of peeling skin on her face and hands was overwhelming. Eventually, she learned that eczema is essentially skin inflammation; a symptom of something deeper. While treatments provided temporary relief, they failed to address the underlying cause. It felt like eczema was a lifelong burden and for years she suffered. Eventually, she decided to delve into the world of holistic health and wellness which taught her that her eczema was just a symptom of deeper inflammation. In Janice's case, she had many food sensitivities and environmental allergies that were all affecting internal and external inflammation; when she started making real changes in her diet and lifestyle, she began to reduce the internal inflammation, and therefore her eczema began to fade; she was able to regulate and predict flare-ups. By understanding her triggers and implementing an anti-inflammatory lifestyle with dietary changes, she embarked on a journey that relieved her of daily pain and discomfort.

Before we delve into how you can make similar changes to fight inflammation, let's take a moment to understand our bodies, particularly our digestive and immune systems, and how inflammation can lead to disease. In this chapter, we'll dive into the gut-inflammation connection and begin the journey toward healing through an anti-inflammatory lifestyle.

The Gut-Inflammation Connection

Our gut is composed of various organs that make up the gastrointestinal system, including the stomach, intestines (both large and small), and colon. Together, these components digest and absorb nutrients from food while eliminating waste. It's a perfectly designed system that supports health when functioning optimally.

Within our gut is a biodiverse ecosystem of bacteria, viruses, and fungi known as the microbiome. These microorganisms break down the food we eat into nutrients that our bodies can absorb and utilize. However, introducing toxins or harmful bacteria can disrupt this balance, potentially leading to various health issues. Gut health is intricately linked to our immune system, and an imbalance in the microbiome can contribute to conditions such as autoimmune disorders, type 2 diabetes, irritable bowel syndrome (IBS), and cardiovascular diseases.

Recognizing signs of an unhealthy gut is crucial. Factors such as chronic stress, fatigue, inadequate sleep, a sedentary lifestyle (see Chapter 3), and poor dietary choices all negatively impact gut health. Some factors may, however, be beyond our control, such as age and early-life experiences like being breastfed versus bottle-fed. But despite these factors, there are steps we can take to support gut health and overall well-being.

Signs of poor gut health may manifest as digestive issues (such as bloating, constipation, or diarrhea), heartburn, sleep disturbances, fatigue, mood swings, high stress levels, and frequent infections. By understanding the gut's vital role in our health and recognizing signs of imbalance, we can arm ourselves with the right tools to support our microbiome and reduce inflammation.

As you already know, inflammation serves a purpose; it's a natural response to something going wrong in our bodies, often in response to a foreign invader. When this occurs, your immune system springs into action, deploying an army of white blood cells (soldiers) to combat the invaders, typically bacteria or viruses. This initial response characterizes acute inflammation. The cells in our gut interact with the microbiome, the community of microorganisms, to fight pathogens and maintain the health of our mucosa.

The mucosa, also known as mucous membrane, is a layer of protective tissue that lines various organs, including the digestive tract. It plays a crucial role in defending against harmful invaders, filtering out toxins, and directing proper nutrient absorption. Essentially, the mucosa acts as a barrier, preventing pathogens from penetrating deeper into the body and causing widespread infection or inflammation.

Seventy to 80% of your immune system is in your digestive tract, where small masses of lymphatic tissue in the small intestine protect the mucous membranes by releasing white blood cells and monitoring the bacteria population. This prevents the overgrowth of harmful bacteria(flora), which can trigger an inflammatory response and compromise the immune system. Chronic illnesses, fueled by inflammation, often stem from imbalances in the gut microbiome and can manifest as symptoms of deeper underlying issues.

A lack of gut biome diversity can lead to inflammation, and low levels of beneficial flora (bacteria) may contribute to conditions such as allergies, eczema, asthma, heart failure, and diabetes. The immune system's response to inflammation can stimulate proteins that promote tumor progression and the onset of type 2 diabetes, as well as increase the risk of cardiovascular diseases. Inflammation, therefore, acts both as a cause and a symptom of various health issues. It's a vicious cycle!

Adding a variety of friendly bacteria to our gut microbiome can offer extra protection and support. This helps promote the growth of beneficial bacteria while keeping harmful pathogens in check, which can improve immune function and reduce inflammation. Eating a diverse range of nutrient-rich foods supports gut health and ensures proper absorption of essential nutrients into our bloodstream. By nourishing our bodies with healthy foods, we can boost immunity and promote overall well-being, ultimately reducing inflammation and improving our overall health.

Fundamentals of Gut Health: Enhancing Gut Health with Simple Strategies

Take in More Probiotics

Probiotics are like the guardians of your gut—they're live bacteria and yeasts that offer many benefits to your body. These friendly bacteria already reside in your body, working alongside many others to maintain balance and support overall health. You'll find probiotics in fermented foods, additionally, you can buy a natural probiotic supplement at most pharmacies, however, natural fermented foods are the healthiest option.

Sources of probiotics include familiar foods like yogurt, kefir, cottage cheese, and miso soup. These nutritious and delicious options not only add variety to your diet but also contribute to the diversity of beneficial bacteria in your gut, the more the merrier, right?

Increase Prebiotics

While probiotics seem to get all the attention, prebiotics are equally important to gut health. Prebiotics are the food source for the beneficial microorganisms in your gut, helping them thrive and flourish. Prebiotics are the favorite food of your healthy bacteria, and when you feed them their favorite food they party and reproduce and act as a gatekeepers by absorbing what your body needs and excluding what it doesn't. Who knew our bodies were designed so well?

Sources of prebiotics include everyday foods like barley, oats, rice, and other high-fiber foods like fruit and vegetables.

Probiotics are the friendly guardians of your gut, fighting off harmful microbes and keeping your digestive system in tip-top shape.

26

They're like the helpful bacteria and yeasts that move into your gut neighborhood, making it a safer and happier place. Then, of course, that means the prebiotics are like the food trucks that roll into town, delivering delicious snacks to these friendly champions. These snacks are essential for keeping the champions strong and energized so they can continue their fight.

In short, probiotics and prebiotics are like the dynamic duo of your gut health, working together to maintain harmony and balance in your digestive system. So, by giving them the right support, you're ensuring that your gut remains a bustling and thriving community of good bacteria.

Hydrate

Hydration is key to maintaining optimal gut health. Adequate water intake is essential for proper nutrient absorption in the digestive system, as water serves as the medium through which nutrients are absorbed into the bloodstream.

For men, it's recommended to drink about 15.5 cups (3.7 liters) of fluids per day, while women should aim for around 11.5 cups (2.7 liters) per day. Of course, it is important to note that individual needs vary based on factors such as physical activity level, climate, and overall health.

Include Gut-Friendly Foods in Your Daily Diet

Eating for gut health doesn't have to be complicated. By incorporating gut-friendly foods into your daily diet, you can feed your microbiome and support overall digestive wellness.

Try these gut-friendly foods:

- Fiber-rich foods:
  - Whole grains like oats and barley
  - Fruits such as bananas, apples, and berries
  - Vegetables like leafy greens, broccoli, and carrots

When it comes to nourishing your gut, there are plenty of delicious options to choose from. Foods rich in fiber are excellent choices. They help promote the growth of beneficial bacteria in your gut, supporting a healthy microbiome.

- Fermented foods:
  - Yogurt
  - Kefir
  - Miso
  - Kimchi

These fermented delights not only add flavor to your dishes but contribute to good gut health by promoting a diverse and thriving microbiome.

- Healthy fats:
  - Avocados
  - Nuts and seeds
  - Olive oil

- Omega-3 fatty acid sources:
  - Fatty fish like salmon and mackerel

These fats help reduce inflammation in the body, which is beneficial for overall digestive function. Including sources of omega-3 fatty acids in your diet, like fatty fish such as salmon or mackerel, can further enhance gut health and reduce the risk of inflammation-related conditions.

- Hydrating foods:
  - Cucumbers
  - Watermelon

Later in this chapter, we'll explore the anti-inflammatory diet in more detail and provide you with a grocery list to help you get started on stocking up with the right foods.

Mindful Eating

Mindful eating is like that friend you never knew you needed until they showed up with a plate of fresh cookies when you're feeling down. We are all busy individuals, and it's easy to overlook the importance of truly savoring our meals. We're often juggling a million things at once, and food sometimes takes a backseat, leaving our bodies and inflammation responses feeling neglected. However, mindful eating habits can save the day and get you on the path toward prioritizing healthy food options all the while enjoying them as well.

Imagine this: you sit down with your meal, take a bite, and instead of mindlessly scarfing it down while scrolling through your phone or binge-watching your favorite show, you take the time to chew slowly and savor each delicious bite. Meal time can be an enjoyable melody of flavors dancing on your pallet, meal after meal.

Food journaling is another tool in the mindful eating toolbox, not a tool for everyone but an option, especially for those who are having inflammation due to food choices in food sensitivities. As someone who has suffered from digestive, inflammation, journalling was a helpful tool for me to understand which foods are fuelling my pains, and which foods ease it. Food journaling was also a helpful tool for me to understand my scheduling when it came to eating and being able to have a better understanding of my habits, choices, preferences, and changes I was making. Becoming more mindful of what I was eating, and how I was eating was one of the largest parts of my healing journey.

But mindful eating doesn't have to be all spreadsheets and calorie counting. It can be as simple as tuning in to your body's signals and stopping when you're full, instead of polishing off that entire pizza just because it tastes so darn good (we've all been there). By reducing distractions and truly focusing on the act of eating, we can forge a deeper connection with our food and our health.

And mindfulness doesn't end when the meal does. Long after we eat we digest, learning to listen and feel this process can also help you have a better understanding of how food is affecting your body. Are you bloated, and gassy or do you feel good and satiated? Take a moment to reflect on how this post-meal check-in can be an important tool in assessing and navigating how food is affecting you without having to write it down or keep a journal. Of course, that's always an option. You can fine-tune your eating habits.

Enjoy your meals more by becoming just a bit more mindful of what you're eating, when you're eating, and reflecting on the results you feel in your body.

Fasting

Eating a healthy whole-food diet makes sense when it comes to healing, but what about not eating? What about fasting? Intermittent fasting has been gaining traction in the health and wellness world, and for good reason. It turns out that giving your gut a break from constant digestion can do wonders for your overall health.

Imagine this: you're on an intermittent fasting journey, and instead of your gut and microbiome disappearing as one might expect, it's doing the opposite. Intermediate fasting can temporarily increase the flourishing of beneficial bacteria in your gut, which helps your immune system function better. Intermediate fasting almost creates a party in your gut. All the good bacteria are invited, and they start reproducing to make more.

Obviously, fasting isn't all rainbows and unicorns! There are some downsides to consider. For starters, you might find yourself feeling a bit hungry (okay, maybe more than a bit) as your body adjusts to the new eating schedule. And let's not forget about the potential dip in energy levels that can accompany fasting. It's like trying to run a marathon with a backpack full of rocks; it's not exactly a walk in the park.

Despite these minor inconveniences, the benefits of intermittent fasting are well worth it. Not only does it promote gut health by increasing microbial diversity, but it also has been shown to reduce inflammation in the body. It's like giving your gut a much-needed vacation, allowing it to rest and recharge so it can come back stronger and healthier than ever. However, our body is reliant on micro and macronutrients, which come from a variety of foods so intermittent fasting is something to consider. However, this is not a long-term or full-time solution. It is something to incorporate into your lifestyle in a way that fits you. Here are some pros and cons of intermittent fasting.

Pros:

- Increases diversity in gut microbiome
- Promotes gut health
- Reduces inflammation in the body
- May aid in weight loss
- Improves insulin sensitivity
- Supports cellular repair processes
- Enhances mental clarity and focus

Cons:

- Hunger during fasting periods
- Potential decrease in energy levels
- Difficulty adhering to fasting schedule
- Possible negative impact on mood
- Risk of overeating during eating windows
- Not suitable for everyone, especially those with certain medical conditions
- Requires careful monitoring and adjustment to find the right fasting routine

So if you're feeling adventurous and are ready to embark on a fasting journey, just remember to listen to your body and take it slow. Start with shorter fasting windows and gradually work your way up as you become more comfortable. And always remember to stay hydrated and nourish your body with nutrient-rich foods during your eating windows. With a little patience and perseverance, you'll be well on your way to reaping the gut-healing benefits of intermittent fasting.

Hippocrates once said, "Let food be thy medicine," and how true is this? Since the most powerful tools in our arsenal to fight inflammation come from the grocery store, the farmers market, and our gardens. It comes from food; eating a diet rich in whole foods. An anti-inflammatory diet is a diet that provides food that feeds our gut microbiome, improves our immunity, and gives us more energy and better quality sleep. An anti-inflammatory diet is a powerful tool in fighting inflammation and promoting overall health. Food truly is medicine, but which foods exactly?

Here are some key components of an anti-inflammatory diet:

1. Antioxidant-Rich Foods: Antioxidants help combat free radicals which contribute to oxidative stress and inflammation in the body. Incorporate plenty of colorful fruits and vegetables such as berries, leafy greens, and bell peppers into your diet. These foods are packed with vitamins, minerals, and phytonutrients that support overall health.

2. High-Fiber Foods: Fiber is essential for gut health and regular bowel movements. Opt for whole grains like oats, quinoa, and brown rice, as well as legumes, nuts, and seeds. These foods help maintain a healthy gut microbiome and promote digestive health.

3. Omega-3 Fatty Acids: Omega-3 fatty acids have powerful anti-inflammatory properties. Include sources of omega-3s such as fatty fish (salmon, mackerel, sardines), flaxseeds, chia seeds, and walnuts in your diet. These fats help reduce inflammation and support heart and brain health.

4. Lean Protein: Protein is essential for tissue repair and muscle growth. Choose lean sources of protein such as poultry, fish, tofu, beans, and lentils. The best results come from whole food proteins like lentils, and beans. Consider adding more of these to your meal planning. These foods provide the building blocks your body needs while minimizing and fighting inflammation.

Foods Contributing to Inflammation

1. Processed Foods: Processed foods are often high in refined sugars, unhealthy fats, and additives that can trigger inflammation in the body. Reduce and or eliminate your intake of processed snacks, sugary beverages, and packaged meals.

2. Refined Carbohydrates: Foods like white bread, white pasta, and sugary cereals are quickly broken down into sugar in the body, leading to spikes in blood sugar levels and inflammation. Opt for whole grains and complex carbohydrates instead.

3. Trans Fats: Trans fats, found in fried foods, baked goods, and margarine, are known to promote inflammation and increase the risk of heart disease. Avoid foods containing hydrogenated oils and opt for healthier fats like olive oil, coconut, nuts, seeds, and avocado.

4. Excessive Alcohol: While moderate alcohol consumption may have some health benefits, excessive drinking can lead to inflammation in the body, especially in the liver. Limit your alcohol intake and stay hydrated with water instead. (see hydration in the previous section)

Controversial Foods

While some foods are known to trigger or worsen inflammation, others have sparked debate within the scientific community due to conflicting research findings. These controversial foods may affect individuals differently, and their inflammatory effects can vary based on factors such as overall diet, genetics, and individual health conditions.

Some of these controversial foods include:

- **Dairy**: While some studies suggest that dairy products may contribute to inflammation, others indicate that certain dairy products like yogurt and kefir containing probiotics may have anti-inflammatory effects.

- **Nightshade vegetables**: Tomatoes, peppers, eggplant, and potatoes are categorized as nightshade vegetables, and some people believe that they can exacerbate inflammation, particularly in individuals with certain autoimmune conditions. However, more research is needed to fully understand their implications on inflammation.

- **Grains**: Gluten-containing grains like wheat, barley, and rye have been implicated in inflammation for individuals with gluten sensitivities or celiac disease. However, for others, whole grains can be part of a balanced anti-inflammatory diet. The healthiest grains are ancient grains like quinoa, amaranth, and farro. These can have positive benefits; however, listen to your body. (See previous section mindful eating)

- **Artificial additives**: Additives such as artificial sweeteners, preservatives, and food dyes found in processed foods and beverages have been linked to inflammation in some studies. However, the direct impact of these additives on inflammation remains a topic of debate among researchers.

It's important to remember that individual responses to these controversial foods can vary, and some individuals may tolerate them well while others may experience increased inflammation. By making mindful choices and focusing on anti-inflammatory foods, you can support your body's natural healing processes and promote overall well-being. Remember, small changes in your diet can make a big difference in how you feel every day. To help you get started below is a grocery list for inspiration.

Anti-Inflammatory Grocery List

Fruits:
- Berries (blueberries, strawberries, raspberries)
- Cherries
- Oranges
- Pineapple
- Apples

- Avocados
- Pomegranates
- Grapes

Vegetables:

- Leafy greens (spinach, kale, Swiss chard)
- Broccoli
- Brussels sprouts
- Bell peppers
- Tomatoes
- Carrots
- Cauliflower
- Sweet potatoes

Whole Grains:

- Quinoa
- Brown rice
- Oats
- Barley
- Whole wheat bread or pasta

Proteins:

- Lentils
- Beans (black beans, kidney beans, chickpeas)
- Tofu
- Tempeh
- Fatty fish (salmon, mackerel, sardines, trout)
- Chicken breast
- Turkey
- Grass-fed beef

Healthy Fats:

- Olive oil
- Nuts (almonds, walnuts, pistachios)
- Seeds (flaxseeds, chia seeds)
- Nut butter (almond butter, peanut butter)

Herbs and Spices:

- Turmeric
- Ginger
- Garlic
- Cinnamon
- Rosemary
- Basil

Beverages:

- Green tea
- Herbal teas (ginger, chamomile)
- Water

Dairy Alternatives:

- Greek yogurt
- Almond milk
- Coconut yogurt

Others:

- Dark chocolate (70% or higher cocoa content)
- Honey
- Fermented foods (sauerkraut, kimchi)

Take your time to reflect on each point and consider how it relates to your personal experiences.

Understand the Gut-Inflammation Connection:

- ☐ Learn how inflammation affects gut health and vice versa.
- ☐ Explore the role of the microbiome in inflammation and overall health.

Fundamentals of Gut Health:

- ☐ Discover the importance of maintaining a healthy gut for overall well-being.
- ☐ Learn about the role of probiotics and prebiotics in supporting gut health.

Probiotics and Prebiotics:

- ☐ Understand what probiotics and prebiotics are and how they benefit gut health.
- ☐ Learn about food sources rich in probiotics and prebiotics.

Stay Hydrated:

- ☐ Recognize the importance of hydration for optimal gut function and overall health.
- ☐ Discover how adequate hydration supports nutrient absorption and digestion.

Mindful Eating:

- ☐ Explore the concept of mindful eating and its benefits for gut health.
- ☐ Learn practical strategies for incorporating mindful eating into daily life.

Gut-Friendly Foods:

- ☐ Identify foods that promote gut health and reduce inflammation.

☐ Discover the benefits of consuming antioxidant-rich, high-fiber, and omega-3-rich foods.

Fasting:

☐ Explore the potential benefits and drawbacks of intermittent fasting for gut health.

☐ Learn about different fasting protocols and their impact on inflammation.

Anti-Inflammatory Eating:

☐ Understand the principles of an anti-inflammatory diet and its role in reducing inflammation.

☐ Discover specific foods and nutrients that support an anti-inflammatory lifestyle.

Controversial Foods:

☐ Learn about foods that may trigger or worsen inflammation in some individuals.

☐ Explore the debate surrounding certain controversial foods and their impact on gut health.

Inflammatory Foods:

☐ Identify common foods that promote inflammation and contribute to gut health issues.

☐ Understand the importance of avoiding or minimizing the consumption of inflammatory foods for optimal health.

How often do you experience digestive discomfort, such as bloating, gas, or indigestion?

1. Never
2. Once in a while
3. A few times a week
4. At least once a day
5. Every meal

Do you consume a diet high in processed foods, sugars, and unhealthy fats?

1. Never
2. Once in a while
3. A few times a week
4. At least once a day
5. Every meal

How frequently do you experience changes in bowel habits, such as constipation or diarrhea?

1. Never
2. Once in a while
3. A few times a week
4. At least once a day

Do you experience symptoms of food intolerances or sensitivities, such as gluten or lactose intolerance?

1. Never
2. Once in a while
3. A few times a week
4. At least once a day
5. Every meal

Are you currently taking any medications that may affect gut health, such as antibiotics or NSAIDs?

1. Never
2. Once in a while
3. A few times a week
4. At least once a day

How would you rate your overall daily stress levels?

1. None
2. Low
3. Moderate
4. Medium to high
5. High

Do you engage in regular physical activity or exercise?

1. At least once a day
2. A few times a week
3. Once in a while
4. Never

How often do you consume probiotic-rich foods, such as yogurt or fermented vegetables?

1. Every meal
2. At least once a day Once in a while
3. A few times a week
4. Once in a while
5. Never

Do you experience symptoms of inflammation, such as joint pain, fatigue, or skin issues?

1. Never
2. Once in a while
3. A few times a week
4. At least once a day

How would you rate your overall energy levels and mood daily?

     1. High energy, positive mood
     3. Moderate energy, occasional fluctuations in mood
     5. Low energy, frequent mood swings

➢ If most of your responses are between 4-5, your diet is most likely a big contributor to your inflammation. Immediate dietary and lifestyle changes are recommended. If your answers vary between 2-3, moderate diet and lifestyle changes are recommended.

Take time to assess your answers and use your responses to help you create an action plan that will help you choose healthier and healing foods.

Now that we've explored how the foods we eat influence inflammation and our overall health, it's time to add another crucial piece to the puzzle: movement. Just as diet plays a significant role in gut health, physical activity and exercise are essential for maintaining optimal digestive function. Let's dive into how movement can support a healthy gut and further enhance our well-being.

Chapter 3 - C.A.**L**.M.N.E.S.S.

L - Leverage Movement to Move Away From Pain

We've talked about the microscopic superheroes working internally to help you heal, but if you think about it you're the driving force for your team. You get to decide if they are at full power or in need of help. You're the team leader, by creating a healthier environment your team (white blood cells) can work harder to repair damage and vanquish invaders (aka viruses, bacteria, and infections). Comprehending was the first step. Feeding your gut what it needs to create a healthy, healing environment was the next step, but as it turns out there is so much more that can be done to continue healing and move away from inflammation for good.

A groundbreaking study from Harvard University reveals the remarkable power of regular exercise to activate immune cells in our muscles, which ultimately can effectively combat inflammation. The study dives into the mechanisms by which physical movement influences our body's inflammatory response. Essentially, when we engage in regular exercise, our muscles release a unique type of immune cell that helps to regulate inflammation throughout the body. Kinda cool, don't you think?

In this chapter, we'll explore how you can harness the healing benefits of exercise and movement to reduce inflammation and pave the way for a more vibrant and pain-free life.

Inflammation can leave us feeling physically weakened, as it gradually erodes our muscles, and tissues, and fuels the onset of diseases, leading to further deterioration. However, there's good news: movement isn't something to fear even in an inflamed state. Recent studies, like the one mentioned, are unveiling the transformative power of physical activity. It's another invaluable tool in our arsenal against inflammation.

When we engage in movement, something remarkable happens: our muscles release proteins, one of which is interleukin-6 (IL-6). This protein plays a crucial role in our body's healing process, particularly in combating chronic inflammation. IL-6 acts as a messenger, signaling the body to initiate the repair and regeneration of damaged tissues. Essentially, it begins a sequence of events that mobilize our body's defenses against inflammation, helping to restore balance and promote overall health.

When you exercise, your body interprets it as a signal that your muscles need repair. This repair process is essential not only for managing inflammation but also for muscle building, toning, and strength development. A recent study from Duke University's biomedical engineers in Durham, NC, confirms that muscle cells possess the ability to regulate inflammation independently under the right conditions.

While it might seem counterintuitive that exercising could worsen inflammation, the opposite is true. When our bodies experience pain or soreness, it's a sign that they're in repair mode. Any effort to enhance this repair process creates a more supportive environment for our body's natural healing mechanisms.

"The doctor of the future will give no medicine, but will involve the patient in the proper use of food, fresh air, and exercise." —
Thomas Edison

Movement is a good thing and nothing to fear!

For those of us who sit at a desk all day, it's easy to feel the results of a sedentary lifestyle, but whether you're sitting at a desk or not spending 6 or more hours sitting, you may be putting yourself at risk for even more inflammation and worse off a list of health problems.

A sedentary lifestyle means sitting or lying down for more than 6 hours a day (on top of your night sleep). Numerous studies show how lack of movement can over time create a toxic internal environment; which can lead to inflammation and can be the fuel that feeds it. Besides contributing to inflammation, lack of physical activity and extended periods of lying down or sitting can reduce and impair your metabolism, your ability to control your blood sugar levels, and inhibit the breakdown of fats, and that's just for starters.

On average each one of us should be engaging in at least 150 minutes of physical exercise each week. About 20 minutes a day. According to a 2017 paper by the Sedentary Behavior Research Network (SBRN), only about 21% of people reach that threshold, while only 5% of people move at least 30 minutes a day. Of course, even if you reach that goal of 20 minutes a day that doesn't get you off the hook even if you spend the rest of the time sitting or lying down. A 15-year study shows that regardless of physical activity if your lifestyle is mainly sedentary, you still increase your chances of early death, as well as a multitude of health issues. A balanced lifestyle of movement is important to heal and maintain health.

Imagine this: Inflammation has set in, so you've reduced your overall movement. You are struggling mentally and physically, but then, all of a sudden, you start feeding yourself amazing healing foods and you start moving your body more… and you know what? You begin to feel better. Your inflammation is reduced and your overall health seems like it's on a path toward healing. This doesn't have to be an imaginary scenario. This can be you; Pain-free, healthy, energetic, and ready to live an extended life. You've already started the first few steps now let's lean into the movement part. What can you do to help you feel better before symptoms progress, other problems, and risk factors increase?

Risks that are associated with the sedentary lifestyle include:

- Heart disease
- High cholesterol
- High blood pressure, hypertension
- Diabetes
- Vein-related problems
- Obesity
- Certain cancers
- Stress, anxiety, and a list of mental issues, including depression

Look, I get it, I've been there. No one wants to think about movement and exercise when they're in pain, but as you know, movement is a helpful healing tool. So let us go through some ways to get you moving so you can activate another tool in your arsenal on your journey toward healing.

Choosing your anti-inflammatory workout

There are plenty of ways to exercise and move your body. However, when you're just getting started, it's best to start slowly, with easy exercises. But before you begin, be sure to set specific goals, because like any new habit, setting goals will help you to reach an overall checkpoint. Results will be different for everyone, depending on your current health status, age, and mobility level. So don't ever compare your goals or progress with anyone else. Some examples of goals might be as simple as walking 5 to 10 minutes each day and leading up to 20 or 30 minutes. Perhaps starting with a few minutes of stretching and breathing every day will lead toward a goal of 20-minute yoga sessions. A few minutes a day sitting on a chair and learning to build strength and resistance with resistance bands; Another great way to get started training yourself toward a larger goal perhaps lifting weights or a physical hobby you've always wanted to try; Like cycling or hiking for example.

- **Walking**: Good for blood circulation and muscle strength while increasing dopamine(that "happy" feeling), especially when you walk outside in nature. Walking has both mental and physical benefits and is a great exercise for beginners.

- **Yoga**: This is described as "meditation in motion" and is an exercise with deep breathing and slow movements. It's a perfect exercise to help reduce blood pressure, and lower anxiety, and depression, not to mention has a positive impact on your overall mental health. Yoga also builds muscle strength and stamina.

- **Body-weight and resistance training**: Both resistance and body-weight training are when you exercise using your body-weight to build strength and muscle. For example, a push-up is a body-weight exercise. You are pushing your entire weight on your arms, which helps build endurance and muscle strength in your arms and shoulders. Resistance bands are often used to help with the external resistance you need for training and building strength. Starting with small amounts of time is the best way for beginners to start. 30 seconds at a time is a good goal to begin with for exercises such as jumping jacks, squats, and bridges.

- **Cycling**: Whether stationary or on the go cycling is a great way to incorporate exercise into your life. Not only is it fun, but you get to set the pace, and a great choice for those who suffer from joint pain and arthritis. It's a low-impact cardiovascular workout that offers many physical and mental health benefits. Not to mention it can be a very pleasurable and enjoyable hobby to do inside or out; however, if you choose to cycle outside in nature, you will experience even more benefits from the positive effects nature has on our overall health.

➢ For best results always do a warm-up before embarking on a short ride. Set small goals like 5-10 minutes to start leading up to a larger goal.

➢ Stretching before any physical activity is recommended especially for beginners

How to kickstart your exercise routine

I'd like to tell you that just moving your body is a great way to get started, and it is, but a little bit of planning goal setting will help you keep on track and move toward goals instead of getting stuck in one spot or lost in your progress. One method for helping you to set goals is by beginning with the S.M.A.R.T. approach, a tool recommended by Harvard Health to help you set goals and keep on track.

S.M.A.R.T. is an acronym for:

S: Specific Goals (goals should have a purpose, what matters right now, and what is the desired result?)

M: Measurable (for example, reaching a weight loss goal that was measured over time)

A: Attainable (realistic for you, what you can do now not what you could do 10 years ago)

R: Relevant (if your goal is to reduce inflammation eating more vegetables every day is a relevant goal)

T: time-bound (Can you make time for this goal right now? Are you giving enough time to reach your goal?)

By following this approach, you can easily begin setting realistic goals for yourself. Remember to break up one larger goal into smaller reachable, attainable goals, slow and steady wins the race. Of course, this is no race. This is a journey toward healing and pain-free toward taming your inflammation for good. So take the time to sit down and think about what you want from your overall healing. What is the ultimate goal and what little steps can you work toward that will make you feel good while heading toward the larger goal?

➢ Tips for getting started:

- Pinpoint your ultimate goal
- Set small, specific mini-goals
- Monitor your progress regularly
- Adapt to changing circumstances
- Don't be hard on yourself

Goal setting example:

Here is someone who wants to build strength, and stamina, and to incorporate cycling into their lifestyle. This example shows the Small weekly goals they aim to reach that are relevant and attainable to their main goal. Regardless of what your overall goal is, consider ways to break that up into smaller goals. Find a way to measure that, and of course, feel free to reward yourself when goals small and large are reached.

Overall Goal: To cycle to the store (35 minutes both ways) without losing my breath or hurting for days afterward

Goal Timeframe: 12 weeks

- **Goal 1 / 2 weeks**: stretching 5 minutes every morning and evening
- **Goal 2 / 2 weeks**: stretching daily 1x, walking 10-15 minutes 2-3 X a week
- **Goal 3 / 2 weeks:** daily stretching, evening walk & cycling 3 X a week 5-10 minutes
- **Goal 4 / 2 weeks:** daily stretching, walking 2-3 evenings 15-20 minutes & cycling to the mailbox 2x a week (10 minutes each way)
- **Goal 5 / 2 weeks:** daily stretching, walking 2-3 X cycle to church 2X (15 minutes each way)
- **Goal 6 / 1 weeks:** daily stretching, walking 2X, cycling to church with a stop at the mailbox 3X (20 minutes each way)
- **12th week.** Ride to the store. Yay! Reward = Buy snacks (Just kidding!). The reward is whatever you want, but the ultimate reward is the feeling of achieving your goal.

Once you've decided on some goals that you're going to work toward it's time to get that butt moving, but fear not this doesn't have to be anything to be scared of. Exercise doesn't have to be daunting or overwhelming exercise, not only helps us toward healing it enhances our mood for an overall more positive self. Exercising can be a very enjoyable experience to incorporate into our lifestyle. Start slow with simple exercises like walking or yoga and try to find ways of including movement in your everyday life beyond exercise and workout routines. Here are some examples of how to move more every day to improve your health, try with simple strategies.

Try these strategies to move more:

- Walk more, in the morning, after supper, to the store. Park farther away, take the stairs, and walk the dog more.
- Do some yoga or stretching every day for a few minutes. Set an alarm every hour to get up, walk around, or stretch especially if you are sitting all day.
- Clean with purpose, bend down to get the baseboards, stand up to fold laundry, dance while you mop or vacuum
- Move while you cook, stand while prepping, stand when taking a call, stand more!
- Try a new physical activity, cycling, rowing, hiking, gardening, or stripping furniture; something you'll enjoy and move your body.
- Play more outside, with your kids, and dogs. Play horseshoes with neighbors, and family pool parties. Spend more time enjoying life outside
- Pump up the jam -I mean put music on, dance while you work, cook, clean, or just dance and feel free. Choose upbeat music that invites you to move
- Stretch or do squats while brushing your teeth, every time you head to the washroom, or open the fridge in between commercials

These strategies will help you move more and feel good while doing it. Of course, having a routine will be great to follow and keep you on track, especially for measuring progress toward specific goals. However, the point is just to get yourself in the habit of moving to get your body used to stretching, flexing, and building stamina so you're consistently sending signals to fight information all the while building up strength for your routine and workout schedules. Life doesn't have to be sedentary. It can be fun and swirling all around us with us in the middle enjoying every moment Instead of watching from the corner of our seat.

Staying on track

We all live busy lives full of obligations, and it can be understandable that there may be some barriers stopping us from getting started, for example:

- Lack of time
- Family obligations
- Low energy
- Low self-confidence
- Fear of injury

These are all reasonable reasons but as the team leader of your body and ultimate health, you are also obligated to yourself to do what you need to feel better. Life is full of obstacles and barriers but you are courageous, strong, smart, and dedicated to your journey of self-healing. There is no lack of time; We can make time! An extra five minutes a day for stretching, and maybe an hour a week for planning healthy meals is not unreasonable. Family is often a difficult obstacle, but at the end of the day you live in your body, it's your vessel, it's your home, and you have to take care of it regardless of other people's opinions, or negativities take charge of your, and step past some of these barriers so you can face the fear that may be holding you back. And of course, it's reasonable to have a fear of hurting yourself. Still, at the end of the day we can hurt ourselves sitting on the couch just as well as we can stretching and lifting weights, so fear the results of not working out rather than the aches and strains, that may result in your efforts and last. Most importantly, you don't judge yourself, everyone falls and fails, what's important is getting up and trying again. You got this! Now wiggle your butt in agreement! ☺

How to get started

- Start with setting goals, and writing them down
- Move more at home and work every day
- Start with short workouts like the ones mentioned in the section above (easy workouts to try)
- Then add in cardio and activities like running, hiking, swimming, etc.
- Stay hydrated and fueled with healthy food
- Invite friends to join you for walks, workouts, yoga classes, or physical activities.
- Stay positive and don't compare yourself to others
- Try a new hobby, gardening, kickboxing, salsa dancing, kayaking, snowshoeing, etc. Have fun moving!
- Don't give up!

Tracking progress

I'll admit that staying motivated can be difficult at times, but that is why tracking your progress is a crucial part of the journey. Remember, dopamine is that "happy" feeling; well, this actually can happen when we acknowledge progress and accomplishments; even more so when we visually see changes like from photos, or tracking journals and data charts. Our brains will register acknowledgment as exciting news which releases dopamine. Positive affirmations and acknowledgment play an important part in staying motivated and energized toward working on your goals. When we feel good and happy we want more of that, it's like chocolate once isn't enough, I want more! Keeping track allows you to visually watch your progress and feel good doing it. But remember, if your progress is slow or not getting better, it's time to switch things up and try something new. More importantly, don't give up or compare yourself to others. Find an accountability partner who has the same goals, and help each other along the road. An accountability partner can provide motivation, support, and a fresh perspective, making the journey to better health more manageable and enjoyable. Plus, you'll be less likely to give up when you don't want to let your partner down.

How to track your progress:

- Keeping track holds you accountable
- Keeps you motivated
- Helps you set realistic goals
- This leads to better results

One of the easiest ways to track your progress is through journaling. You can do this with a notebook or on your phone, and of course, there are tons of free fitness apps that you can use to help you keep track. To get started with journaling try using some of these prompts.

- What exercise did you do?
- How many reps, steps, miles, etc?
- How long did you exercise?
- What time of day was it?
- Where did you exercise?
- Did you eat before and or after?
- Did you reach a milestone or a personal best?
- How did you feel physically, mentally, and emotionally during, before, and after your workout?

These are just a guide to help you get started feel free to personalize these questions or leave some unanswered whenever it's relevant.

The exercise- Inflammation Equation

- ☐ Learn how regular physical activity combats chronic inflammation.
- ☐ Discover the role of muscle cells and the IL-6 protein in fighting inflammation.
- ☐ Explore evidence and studies highlighting the anti-inflammatory effects of exercise.

Awareness of Sedentary Lifestyle Dangers

- ☐ Define a sedentary lifestyle and its associated health risks.
- ☐ Recognize the implications of prolonged sitting on various aspects of health, from vein-related problems to increased stress levels.

Selecting Anti-Inflammatory Workouts:

- ☐ Identify different types of exercises effective in reducing inflammation, including walking, yoga, bodyweight exercises, mobility exercises, and cycling.
- ☐ Understand the benefits of each type of exercise in combating inflammation.

Initiating Your Exercise Routine:

- ☐ Incorporate simple strategies to add more movement into daily life, such as going for walks, doing yoga or stretching, and taking the stairs.
- ☐ Set achievable goals for exercise, focusing on specific mini-goals and monitoring progress regularly.

Overcoming Exercise Barriers:

- ☐ Address common barriers to regular exercise, including lack of time, family obligations, and low energy.
- ☐ Discover motivational tips to stay on track, including

starting with short workouts, inviting a friend to join, and not comparing oneself to others.

Maintaining Motivation through Progress Tracking:

- ☐ Understand the importance of tracking progress in maintaining motivation and accountability.
- ☐ Learn how progress tracking triggers dopamine release in the brain, reinforcing positive behaviors and improvements in health and fitness.

Fitness Self-Assessment Quiz:

Take your time to answer each question honestly. Your responses will help you understand your current fitness status and guide you in setting appropriate fitness goals.

1. Cardiovascular Endurance:

How would you rate your ability to sustain aerobic activities, such as running, swimming, or cycling?

1: Very poor
2: Poor
3: Average
4: Good
5: Excellent

2. Muscular Strength:

How would you rate your overall strength and ability to perform resistance exercises?

1: Very weak
2: Weak
3: Average
4: Strong
5: Very strong

3. Flexibility:

How would you rate your flexibility and range of motion in your joints?

1: Very limited
2: Limited
3: Average
4: Good
5: Excellent

4. Balance and Stability:

How confident do you feel in maintaining balance during various activities?

1: Very unsteady
2: Unsteady
3: Average
4: Stable
5: Very stable

5. Core Strength:

How strong do you feel your core muscles are in supporting your spine and maintaining good posture?

1: Very weak
2: Weak
3: Average
4: Strong
5: Very strong

6. Overall Fitness Level:

Considering all aspects of fitness, how would you rate your current fitness level?

1: Very poor
2: Poor
3: Average
4: Good
5: Excellent

If you answered with more 1s and 2s:

Your fitness level may need significant improvement in various areas such as cardiovascular endurance, muscular strength, flexibility, balance, stability, and core strength. Consider starting with low-intensity exercises and gradually increasing intensity and duration to build overall fitness.

If you answered with more 3s:

Your fitness level is moderate, showing that you have a decent foundation in areas such as cardiovascular endurance, muscular strength, flexibility, balance, stability, and core strength. To continue progressing, consider incorporating a mix of moderate-intensity exercises and gradually introducing higher-intensity workouts. This balanced approach will help you improve your overall fitness while avoiding potential plateaus.

If you answered with more 4s and 5s:

Your fitness level indicates good to excellent performance across multiple areas, including cardiovascular endurance, muscular strength, flexibility, balance, stability, and core strength. Focus on maintaining your current fitness level and consider setting new challenges to further enhance your overall performance.

Having delved into the transformative role of diet and exercise in managing inflammation, it's essential to shine a spotlight on another significant player in the inflammation narrative: stress. Let's head to Chapter 4 and learn how stress plays a role in our body.

Chapter 4 - C.A.L.**M**.N.E.S.S.

M - Managing Stress

We've all heard the saying "stress is a killer" and the horrible truth is, it's true! Stress is the ultimate villain and the root of evil for at least six major causes of death. Eeek! Scary, right? But rest assured, because we are on a healing journey toward the whole self; Mind, body, and ultimately soul. As we embark on this journey toward comprehensive self-healing, we can see we are on a holistic path, a more natural route. From our road to understanding, eating healthier, and moving more, we can now take on the next step: managing stress.

Everyone has stress, it's a normal and natural part of living. Stress is simply a response to a new and challenging or threatening situation. Just like our body reacts to infection or wear and tear, our bodies also respond to stressful situations, which then trigger stress hormones. If stress is ongoing and becomes overwhelming, it can lead to chronic stress and when the word "chronic" comes into play, we know it's not a good thing. Chronic stress can lead to mental and physical health problems; anxiety, pain, depression, and so much more.

As I mentioned earlier, stress is a killer because chronic stress can deteriorate our bodies and minds. Even worse, stress can worsen other conditions like inflammation.

Let's explore stress in this chapter and learn how to manage it in ways that best fit your lifestyle. Stress is normal; how we handle it makes all the difference.

Picture this: You have a big presentation tomorrow and your computer just crashed, causing you to lose all your files. You panic and frantically try to recover the files from your computer, trying everything you can, even becoming a little aggressive and agitated. This leads you to fall behind and so you are unable to prepare anything for your presentation. You find yourself unable to sleep, and a headache follows for days. A new lack of confidence begins to show in your work.

Now, imagine a scenario where your reaction was different. Instead of trying to fix the problem you know you can't solve because you're not a computer engineer, you turn to your colleagues and ask for advice. Together, you collaborate to try and re-create notes and charts you had previously prepared on your computer. That way, when you walk into your meeting tomorrow, you have something to present. aYou can feel confident knowing that you did your best to resolve the issue to the best of your ability. You feel good attacking the problem head-on, rather than running from it.

With a clear mind, you were able to remember most of the presentation, and overall, despite the technical issues, you did a good job. This gives you a well-deserved boost in confidence and maybe even a reward, like, hmmm... Takeout and an early bedtime?

Unfortunately, stress can't be the beginning of a ball no one wants to chase down the hill. How we react to stress will determine the results on our body and mind. Temporary or short-term stress is not a bad thing. It's healthy for us to have stress, it helps us to perceive threats or dangers, and it's just another mechanism for our body to protect itself. When we encounter a challenge or danger, stress releases hormones that increase our fight-or-flight reaction. Our heart rate and blood pressure go up, giving us a boost of energy to face the problem. However, when stress builds up and becomes overwhelming, it can lead to chronic stress if untreated. Ignoring or mishandling stress can impact your physical and mental health daily and cause long-term chronic conditions. Additionally, it can worsen issues like inflammation.

Signs of chronic stress may include at least two of these symptoms:

- Mood swings
- Insomnia, restless sleep
- Fatigue, tired all the time
- Weight changes, weight loss, and/or weight gain
- Digestion issues
- Impatient and irritability
- Unable to concentrate and disorganized thoughts
- Headaches
- Anxiety and panic attacks
- Depression
- Increased tension in your body
- New or heightened, obsessive behavior, compulsive behavior

The Stress-Inflammation Connection

When we face acute stress, our body releases hormones to help us respond. However, prolonged stress leads to continuous hormone release, which stimulates the production of pro-inflammatory substances called cytokines. If these hormones persist, they trigger an inflammatory response or worsen existing inflammation.

When you're stressed, hormones like cortisol are released to suppress nonessential functions, such as your immune response and digestion. These hormones are part of the fight-or-flight response. Cortisol boosts glucose production to increase energy, but it also reduces insulin production, which can narrow your arteries.

Another hormone released when you are stressed is adrenaline. This hormone signals the body to expand the airways and push more oxygen, which results in increased heart and respiratory rates. Together these mechanisms help us respond to short-term stress. When you're stressed, your body produces fewer lymphocytes, which are white blood cells crucial for your immune system. This reduction increases your risk of viral infections, such as the common cold.

Constantly living in a heightened state of stress puts a strain on your body's overall functions, making it harder for your body to heal and maintain a healthy environment.

Chronic conditions linked to stress

According to the American Psychological Association (APA), 67% of Americans have reported feeling more stressed since 2020. This increase in stress is likely due to the height of the COVID-19 pandemic, which was a particularly stressful time. Believe it or not, for some people that stress is still ongoing, lingering, and has become chronic.

No matter what the situation is that triggers stress, when stress isn't managed properly, it can lead to some serious diseases. Here are some of these diseases directly related to chronic stress:

- Rheumatoid arthritis (RA), which is directly related to the overproduction of Cytokines, is the result of ongoing stress. What's worse, RA can lead to more serious problems like heart attacks, stroke, or even cancer.

- IBD is an inflamed bowel disease. Stress can cause many gastrointestinal issues such as Crohn's.

- Depression: Hormone imbalances induced by stress can affect the brain's immune cell activation causing depression or anxiety responses. Inflammation can also lead to symptoms that look like depression in people who are already in a depressed state

Navigating stress with practical solutions

Stress is kind of scary, wouldn't you agree? But not unmanageable! I'm sure you probably know someone who always seems happy, keeps themselves busy, and is never stressed out. It's not that they don't have stress. I mean we all do! However, usually, these individuals have learned how to navigate daily stresses better than you, so life seems easier and in some cases happier. These individuals often find time for hobbies and interests, and they make self-care a priority—and I don't mean makeup and nails. Perhaps they exercise, eat right, meditate, or all three. Whatever skills or habits they have to help them cope with the day-to-day you can have them too. Trying different strategies is the best way to help you figure out how to navigate and manage your stress. Let us go through some benefits of stress management and strategies to try.

Benefits of stress management

Learning to manage stress offers numerous benefits. It enhances your problem-solving abilities and internal functioning. Lower stress levels lead to a healthier immune system and overall better health. Remember, you're in charge of creating a positive environment for your body's internal systems to thrive. Other advantages include maintaining a healthy weight more easily, enjoying better sleep, experiencing improved mood and clearer thinking, and nurturing better relationships in all aspects of life. By mastering stress management techniques, you're also helping to prevent major diseases and reduce overall inflammation. Moreover, effective stress management provides the energy and motivation necessary to continue on your healing journey. Remember, the goal of this journey is to shift away from survival mode and toward a life that's easier to enjoy and experience fully.

Practicing Relaxation techniques to help reduce stress can:
- Slow heart rate
- Lower blood pressure
- Slow breathing rate
- Improve digestion
- Control blood sugar levels
- Lessened activity of stress hormones
- Increase blood flow to major muscles
- Ease muscle tension and chronic pain
- Improve focus and mood
- Improve sleep quality
- Lower fatigue

- Lessen anger and frustration
- Boost confidence to handle problems

Want to know how to relax and stay mindful? We'll dive into relaxation and mindfulness methods later in the chapter, but first, let's discuss some techniques that help you manage your stress levels.

Strategies to try for everyday situations

- **Speak up for yourself.** Communication is an important part of dealing with stressful situations, relationships, and problems. Expressing your thoughts and feelings clearly can help resolve issues more effectively and reduce misunderstandings, leading to less stress and better outcomes in your interactions.

- **Take action to solve the problem.** Find another route or do something different. Don't just ignore the issue or allow the situation to repeat. Addressing the problem head-on can prevent it from happening again and help you feel more in control.

- **Get organized at home, at your office, and in your car.** Having a tidy space helps you stay organized internally, leading to fewer scattered thoughts. This can also help you take quick action when faced with stressful situations.

- **Creating your own space** is essential for managing stress effectively. This space serves as a sanctuary where you can retreat to find solitude and tranquility. Whether you use it for reading, pursuing hobbies, listening to music, or simply sitting quietly to clear your mind or engage in problem-solving, having your own designated area can significantly contribute to your overall well-being. It provides a sense of sanctuary and refuge from the demands and stresses of everyday life, allowing you to recharge and rejuvenate. This space can be as simple as a cozy corner in your home or a designated room where you can unwind and decompress. By carving out this space for yourself, you're creating a physical and mental environment that supports relaxation and inner peace, essential elements of effective stress management.

- **Understanding expectations** is crucial for maintaining harmonious relationships and effective communication. Take the time to clarify expectations with your partner at home, your children, and your colleagues at work. When everyone involved has a clear understanding of what is expected of them, it becomes much easier to navigate relationships, collaborate on projects, and address any potential conflicts. Effective communication ensures that everyone is on the same page, reducing the likelihood of misunderstandings or disagreements. It's important to remember that this understanding works both ways—make sure to seek clarification from your partner, coworkers, and friends about their expectations as well. By fostering an environment of open communication and mutual understanding, you can cultivate stronger and more supportive relationships in all areas of your life.

- **Avoid multitasking when possible**, this can be super stressful for a lot of people creating disorganization and chaos when in a heightened or stressful situation, place, or relationship. Focus on one thing at a time whenever possible. This will help you keep your stress levels down and address stress as it happens.

- **Be comfortable** whether you're at work, at home, or with family. You should be able to be yourself and feel at ease in any environment. Whether that means being comfortable in the clothing you're wearing, or comfortable to safely speak your mind, you shouldn't feel like you're walking on eggshells, or having to hide or lie. This can cause high stress and make stress management difficult. Sometimes etiquette and formality are required. Still, do your best to feel as comfortable as you can in your skin, your voice, your own space, and with the people you're spending time with.

- **Remove external stresses.** This is easier said than done, however, sometimes removing people from our lives, avoiding certain places, changing habits, and so forth can be the easiest way to avoid certain stresses

- **Self-care in the moment of stress**, try taking a walk, doing deep breathing exercises, making herbal tea, listening to music, or doing something fun. Try to find some humor and positivity in a stressed moment to help reduce, or avoid an emotional escalation.

- **Exercise** is proven to enhance your mood, regular exercise will help reduce stress levels and help you navigate easier during stressful moments. As discussed, movement is a powerful tool in fighting inflammation and stress too.

- **Eat well.** Food is medicine for the body and mind. As you know this is the ultimate tool and maintaining a healthy diet will help you reduce stress just like exercising will help you navigate easier doing stressful situations

- **Mindfulness** (are you noticing a pattern yet?) involves thinking before you communicate or react, taking time to assess your thoughts, and learning how to relax your mind. Practicing mindfulness helps you understand yourself better, including how you communicate and respond to situations. One of the best ways to learn mindfulness is by trying relaxation techniques such as meditation.

Imagine this: You ordered a new piece of furniture for guests arriving in a couple of days. As you unbox it, you realize it's missing the essential tool needed for assembly. Before practicing mindfulness, you might have panicked, torn apart all the packages, lost or damaged pieces, and then angrily called customer service to complain. But not now. On your healing journey, you're eating a healthy diet, exercising regularly, and learning to manage stress.

You take a deep breath. Instead of getting angry and taking it out on the customer service person, you take a moment to assess the situation. You walk across the street and, without expectation, ask your neighbor if they have the tool you need. Not only does your neighbor have the tool, but they also offer to help you assemble the furniture.

What could have been a stressful situation turned into a simple problem-solving exercise. By taking a moment to breathe and think, you not only solved the problem but made the process much easier.

Learning to manage your time effectively is vital for reducing stress because it empowers you to prioritize tasks, avoid procrastination, and maintain a healthy balance between work and personal life. Here are some benefits of learning to manage your time better:

- Prioritization - When you manage your time well, you can identify and tackle important tasks first, helping you avoid feeling overwhelmed by a long to-do list.

- Reduced Procrastination - Effective time management breaks tasks into manageable chunks, reducing the urge to procrastinate and the stress that comes with looming deadlines.

- Increased Productivity - By staying focused and organized, you'll accomplish more in less time, leading to a greater sense of accomplishment and less stress from unfinished work.

- Better Work-Life Balance - Managing your time allows you to allocate time for both work and personal activities, helping you avoid burnout and maintain overall well-being.

- Sense of Control - When you're in control of your schedule, you'll feel less overwhelmed by external pressures and more confident in your ability to handle challenges effectively.

Here are some effective time management techniques to help you reduce stress:

- Prioritize tasks: Identify the most important tasks and tackle them first.
- Break tasks into smaller steps: Divide larger tasks into smaller, more manageable chunks to prevent overwhelm.
- Set deadlines: Establish deadlines for tasks to maintain focus and motivation.
- Use a calendar or planner: Keep track of deadlines, appointments, and commitments to stay organized.
- Limit multitasking: Focus on one task at a time to improve

productivity and reduce stress.

- Set realistic goals: Set achievable goals to prevent feelings of failure and stress.
- Take regular breaks: Schedule short breaks throughout the day to recharge and prevent burnout.
- Delegate tasks: Delegate tasks when possible to lighten your workload and free up time for other priorities.
- Learn to say no: Set boundaries and prioritize your own needs by saying no to tasks or commitments that don't align with your goals.
- Practice the Pomodoro Technique: Work in focused intervals (e.g., 25 minutes of work followed by a 5-minute break) to maintain productivity and avoid burnout.

Remember the importance of scheduling downtime amidst your busy days. Taking mental breaks, where you're not actively problem-solving or learning, can significantly enhance your mood, performance, and ability to concentrate. Embrace moments of stillness and relaxation, as they offer vital opportunities for rejuvenation and mental clarity, ultimately contributing to a more balanced and stress-free life.

The role of mindfulness and relaxation

Mindfulness is the practice of focusing your awareness on the present moment, over and over again, as well as on sensations that route you into your body in the here and now.

In a 2021 study published in the Frontiers in Psychology, people who participated in a six-week mindfulness course reported lower stress levels.

Similarly, a 2019 study in the same journal found that mindfulness meditation helped improve depression and anxiety symptoms, partly by reducing worry and rumination (thinking about something over and over and over again). A 2022 randomized clinical trial published in JAMA Psychiatry found mindfulness-based stress reduction to be just as effective as escitalopram, an SSRI that's a first-line prescription medication for anxiety and depression. However, it's important to note that this doesn't mean that mindfulness is the cure or solution for all people and all cases of anxiety and depression. It simply highlights the potential effectiveness of mindfulness-based approaches, and an option to consider for your treatment and healing efforts.

The mind is adept at problem-solving and navigating the past and future, but being present in the moment is a skill that requires practice. Regular practice makes dealing with everyday situations, especially stressful ones, easier. Here are some tips to begin practicing mindfulness and relaxation techniques, all of which involve focusing on one thing at a time, whether it's yourself, your breath, an external sound, or a visual.

- **Three-minute breathing space** - Find a quiet space to retreat to your own space, and set a timer for three minutes while sitting in a comfortable position. Bring your full attention to your breath, focusing on the sensation of the air flowing in and out of your body. Expand your awareness further out from your breathing so that it includes your whole body. You might notice your posture, your facial expression, or areas of muscle tension. Again, simply pay attention to whatever's going on with your body. And breathe.

- **Mindful listening** - Focusing on a specific sound no matter where you are, traffic in the distance, the sound of a squeak on the bus, or the hum of a fan in a room next door. Try to focus on one specific sound and think about how it resonates. Does it have a pattern of a low tone or high tone, pick out a sound, and just listen to it!

- **Body scan** - Focusing on your body, usually starting down at your feet, working your way up, and focusing on the sensations and feelings as you scan your way to the top.

- **4-7-8 mindful breathing** - Inhale for four seconds hold for seven exhale for eight. This is a great exercise for anxiety. It helps concentrate your breathing and lower your heart rate.

- **People-watching** - This is a great way to detach from yourself and focus your mind on others around you. Whether you're on a walk, at work, or sitting on your front porch, observe how people walk and look. Remember, the goal is to engage in a mindful activity without being judgmental or critical. If you don't feel comfortable watching people, observing animals and pets is also a good option.

Other relaxation techniques to try

- **Autogenic relaxation:** This technique involves focusing inward to promote a state of deep relaxation. Start by visualizing a peaceful place or a calming memory that makes you feel safe and serene. Once you have this image in your mind, shift your focus to your breath. Take slow, deep breaths, feeling the rise and fall of your chest with each inhale and exhale. As you continue to breathe deeply, direct your attention to your heart rate. Imagine it slowing down, beating in a calm, steady rhythm. By combining these elements— peaceful imagery, controlled breathing, and heart rate awareness— you can achieve a state of relaxation that helps reduce stress and promotes overall well-being.

- **Progressive muscle relaxation:** This technique involves tensing and then relaxing each muscle group in your body to promote deep relaxation and release tension. Begin by focusing on one muscle group at a time. For example, start with your toes—tense the muscles as tightly as you can for about five seconds. Then, release the tension and relax the muscles completely for about 30 seconds. Move progressively through the rest of your body, working up from your feet to your head. As you do this, pay attention to the contrast between the feeling of tension and the sensation of relaxation, allowing yourself to experience a deep sense of calm and relief throughout your entire body.

- **Visualization:** This technique involves creating a vivid mental image to transport yourself to a calming place. Begin by choosing a serene location, such as a beach. Close your eyes and immerse yourself in this mental journey. Picture the ocean vividly—see the waves, imagine the sparkling water, and visualize the sun warming your skin. Engage all your senses: smell the salty sea air, feel the sand beneath your feet, and hear the soothing sound of waves crashing on the shore. By fully engaging all your senses in this focused visualization, you can create a profound sense of relaxation and escape from stress.

- **Deep breathing exercises**: Deep breathing is a form of meditation that helps promote relaxation and focus. There are several techniques you can use. For example, you might count your breaths from 1 to 4, paying close attention to the sensation and sound of each inhale and exhale. Focus on how the breath feels as it enters and leaves your body.

- **Guided meditation**: Another effective method for beginners is guided meditation, which provides structured instructions to help you get started and maintain focus. This can be a helpful way to learn deep breathing techniques and integrate them into your relaxation practice.

- **Massage:** Visiting a professional masseuse or receiving a massage from a loved one is a wonderful way to release muscle tension and promote relaxation. Regular massages can help alleviate stress, ease muscle soreness, and enhance overall well-being. Whether you schedule sessions with a professional or enjoy a relaxing massage at home, incorporating this practice into your routine can significantly contribute to reducing stress and improving your sense of calm.

- **Yoga**: Yoga combines meditation with physical movement, creating a practice that integrates both mind and body. It involves slow, deliberate exercises and controlled breathing techniques designed to enhance flexibility, strength, and relaxation. Through a series of poses and mindful breathing, yoga helps calm the mind, reduce stress, and improve overall physical and mental well-being.

- **Tai Chi:** Tai Chi is an ancient Chinese martial art known for its slow, flowing movements and focus on deep breathing. Similar to yoga, it emphasizes gentle, deliberate motion combined with mindful breathing to enhance balance, flexibility, and relaxation. Practicing Tai Chi can help reduce stress, improve mental clarity, and promote overall well-being through its meditative and rhythmic approach.

- **Music, Art, or Garden Therapy**: Engaging in activities like music, art, or gardening can be deeply therapeutic when done in a meditative state. By focusing fully on these activities, you immerse yourself in the present moment, which can enhance self-awareness and relaxation. Whether you're playing an instrument, painting, or tending to plants, combining your hobbies with mindful practice offers numerous mental and physical benefits. These activities help reduce stress, improve mood, and foster a greater sense of well-being.

- **Aromatherapy**: Aromatherapy involves using essential oils derived from herbs and plants to promote relaxation and well-being. These oils can be diffused into the air, applied to the skin, or used in steam or smoke. Different herbs have varying properties—some are calming and healing, while others have medicinal benefits. Research indicates that inhaling certain fragrances can directly affect the brain, helping to reduce stress and anxiety. By incorporating aromatherapy into your routine, you can harness these scents to enhance your overall sense of calm and mental clarity.

- **Hydrotherapy:** Hydrotherapy utilizes water in various forms, such as baths, showers, wraps, and compresses, to provide therapeutic effects. For example, soaking in a warm bath can help relax muscles and joints, while cold water immersion can reduce inflammation and numb pain. Additionally, water pressure from jets in a spa or whirlpool can provide massage-like benefits to improve circulation and reduce tension. Overall, the use of water in hydrotherapy helps to stimulate the body's natural healing processes and promote overall well-being.

Most of these strategies for stress management are simple and easy to try. Let's be honest, we could all benefit from better stress management. Experiment with these natural and straightforward methods to see which one works best for you and helps you feel more at ease.

Don't forget to jot down your thoughts and observations as you go through the checklist!

Understand the signs and sources of stress in your life:

☐ Recognize common stressors, such as work deadlines, financial concerns, or relationship issues.

☐ Identify physical symptoms of stress, including muscle tension, headaches, and changes in appetite or sleep patterns.

☐ Acknowledge emotional signs of stress, such as irritability, anxiety, or feelings of overwhelm.

Learn and apply practical strategies to manage your stress effectively:

☐ Explore a variety of stress management techniques, including deep-breathing exercises, mindfulness meditation, and progressive muscle relaxation.

☐ Develop healthy coping mechanisms to deal with stressors, such as maintaining a support network, setting realistic goals, and practicing self-compassion.

☐ Incorporate stress-reducing activities into your daily routine, such as spending time in nature, engaging in hobbies, or practicing gratitude.

Incorporate time management techniques into your daily routines:

☐ Prioritize tasks based on importance and urgency to minimize feelings of overwhelm.

☐ Use tools such as to-do lists, calendars, and time-blocking techniques to organize your schedule and manage your time effectively.

☐ Set boundaries and learn to say no to tasks or commitments that contribute to stress or overload.

Practice mindfulness and relaxation exercises to lower your stress levels:

- ☐ Cultivate present-moment awareness through mindfulness practices such as mindful breathing, body scans, or mindful eating.
- ☐ Engage in relaxation techniques such as guided imagery, progressive muscle relaxation, or visualization to reduce muscle tension and promote relaxation.
- ☐ Incorporate mindfulness into daily activities, such as mindful walking, mindful listening, or mindful communication with others.

Develop resilience and coping skills to navigate challenging situations in your life:

- ✱ ☐ Cultivate a growth mindset and view challenges as opportunities for learning and growth.
- ☐ Foster social connections and seek support from friends, family, or mental health professionals during times of stress.
- ☐ Practice self-care activities such as exercise, adequate sleep, healthy nutrition, and leisure activities to recharge and replenish your energy.

Self-assessment

1. How often do you experience stress-related symptoms, such as irritability, fatigue, or headaches?

1. Never
2. Rarely
3. Occasionally
4. Frequently
5. Daily

2. Do you find it challenging to relax and unwind after a stressful day?

1. Never
2. Rarely
3. Occasionally
4. Frequently
5. Always

3. How well do you cope with unexpected stressors or changes in your routine?

1. Very well
2. Moderately well
3. Neutral
4. Not very well
5. Poorly

4. Can you maintain a healthy work-life balance, or do you often feel overwhelmed by work or personal responsibilities?

1. I have a healthy balance
2. I sometimes feel overwhelmed
3. I frequently feel overwhelmed
4. I often feel overwhelmed
5. I always feel overwhelmed

5. How often do you practice relaxation techniques, such as deep breathing, meditation, or mindfulness?

1. Daily
2. Several times a week
3. Once a week
4. Rarely
5. Never

6. Do you have a support system or social network that you can turn to during times of stress?

1. Strong support system
2. Moderate support system

3. Limited support system
4. Minimal support system
5. No support system

7. How effectively do you manage your time and prioritize tasks to reduce stress?

1. Very effectively
2. Moderately effectively
3. Neutral
4. Not very effectively
5. Not at all effectively

8. Are you able to identify and address the sources of your stress proactively?

1. Always
2. Often
3. Sometimes
4. Rarely
5. Never

9. How often do you engage in physical activity or exercise to help manage stress?

1. Daily
2. Several times a week
3. Once a week
4. Rarely
5. Never

10. How would you rate your overall stress levels on a scale of 1 to 5, with 1 being minimal stress and 5 being extreme stress?

1. Minimal stress
2. Low stress
3. Moderate Stress
4. High stress
5. Extreme stress

Assess your scores

- If you scored mostly "1" and "2": You are effectively managing stress and using healthy coping strategies. Keep up the good work! To maintain this positive momentum, continue practicing your current techniques and consider exploring new methods to further enhance your resilience.

- If you scored mostly "3" and "4": Consider incorporating additional stress management techniques and seeking support if needed to enhance your coping skills. Reflect on your current strategies and identify areas where you can improve or add new approaches to better manage stress.

- If you scored mostly "5": Focus on prioritizing self-care and stress reduction practices to better manage your stress levels and improve your overall well-being. Additionally, consider reaching out for professional help to address underlying issues and receive tailored support.

Now that we have a better understanding of stress, its effects, and how to manage it, it's time to consider another crucial aspect of well-being: sleep. Just as stress can influence inflammation levels, inadequate or poor-quality sleep can worsen inflammation in the body. Let's look into how optimizing your sleep patterns can support your journey to combat chronic inflammation and enhance overall health and vitality.

Chapter 5 - C.A.L.M.**N**.E.S.S.

N - Nurturing Sleep

What if I told you that the quality of your sleep can directly affect the DNA responsible for your immune system's ability to defend against infection and disease? It might sound surprising, but research from Mount Sinai reveals just how vital sleep is for our overall health. In a groundbreaking study, a mere 90-minute reduction in sleep led to significant changes in immune cells and alterations in DNA structure. Even more astonishing is that these changes persisted even after sleep was recovered, indicating ongoing stress to the body. This persistent stress increases the production of white blood cells, thereby elevating the risk of inflammation and worsening existing conditions.

Humans, as well as most animals, have a natural process that regulates the wake-sleep cycle known as the circadian rhythm. This intricate system involves interactions between the central nervous system, endocrine system, and immune system to maintain our sleep-wake cycle. Disrupting this natural rhythm interferes with the body's essential repair mechanisms. Sleep isn't just a luxury; it's a crucial element in your toolkit for combating chronic inflammation.

The Science of Sleep

Human sleep is divided into four stages: the first three are non-REM (rapid eye movement) sleep, and the fourth is REM sleep. Each sleep cycle typically lasts around 90 minutes, but the duration of each stage can vary. REM sleep usually becomes more prominent as the night progresses, and the patterns shift throughout the night. Disruptions or shortened sleep can interrupt the natural flow of these stages, affecting the overall quality of rest. Factors such as age, recent sleep patterns, and alcohol consumption can also impact sleep patterns. The time spent in each stage can differ from person to person. Let's explore these stages and patterns in more detail to better understand how the body functions during sleep.

The 4 stages of sleep are Non-REM sleep 1-3 N.1, N.2, N.3, and REM sleep.

1. **Stage 1: N.1** is the first cycle in which your body and brain attempt to reach a relaxed and slowed state. During N.1 you are not fully relaxed and you can easily be woken up. However, if undisturbed within 1-7 minutes you can reach stage 2 in the sleep cycle.

2. **Stage 2: N.2** is the next cycle where your brain begins to fall into a subdued state and your body temperature slightly lowers. Your muscles reach a relaxed state and your breathing and heart rate are slowed.

3. **Stage 3: N.3** is deep sleep, a phase where waking up becomes much more difficult. During this stage, muscle tone, pulse, and breathing rate decrease, leaving you in a profoundly relaxed state. Your brain waves slow down to delta patterns, which is why this stage is also known as delta sleep. This period is crucial for restorative processes, including recovery and growth. Research shows that deep sleep supports insightful thinking, creativity, and memory consolidation.

4. **Stage 4: REM sleep** - During REM (rapid eye movement) sleep, your brain is highly active, almost as much as when you're awake. It's busy processing emotions, reinforcing memories, and supporting learning and creativity. This stage is crucial for mental and emotional health. During REM sleep, your breathing becomes faster and irregular, and your voluntary muscles are temporarily paralyzed to prevent you from acting out your dreams. This is when you experience the most vivid dreams.

All stages of sleep are essential for health and healing. Throughout the night, our body and brain cycle through these stages multiple times. REM sleep typically occurs only after completing about 90 minutes of N.2 and N.3 sleep cycles.

Stages 3 and REM (Stage 4) are vital for healing and growth. During these deep sleep stages, our bodies produce hormones that support bone and muscle growth, enhance immune function, and facilitate repair and rebuilding. To effectively address symptoms of illness or injury, or in other words, to combat inflammation, getting sufficient sleep is crucial.

Each stage of sleep plays a critical role in different recovery processes for our body and brain. When we don't get enough sleep or experience disrupted sleep, the effects can be serious and long-lasting, impacting both our short-term well-being and long-term health.

A lack of or disrupted sleep can lead to:
- Learning and focus problems
- Increased risk of mood swings, anxiety, and depression
- Lack of creativity
- Hard to make rational decisions
- Difficulty problem solving
- Recalling information and memories
- Confrontational, hard-to-control emotions and behavior

Failure to reach sleep stages can also put you at risk for these conditions:
- Pain and inflammation disorders and symptoms
- High blood pressure
- Heart disease
- Higher production of stress hormones
- Overweight and obesity
- Metabolic disorders
- Diabetes
- Low quality of life

Getting enough sleep regularly will greatly improve your life and be just another tool in your arsenal to heal and combat pain.

Role of sleep in combating inflammation

During sleep, your body carries out crucial processes to repair and rejuvenate itself, including managing inflammation. A key player in this process is cytokines—small proteins vital for coordinating immune responses. Think of them as the dedicated foot soldiers of your immune system, working tirelessly to maintain your health and protect you. While you sleep, your body ramps up cytokine production to help regulate inflammation and fight off infections.

However, when you don't get enough sleep, this balance can be disrupted. Studies have shown that sleep deprivation leads to decreased cytokine production, making you more vulnerable to inflammation and infections. Just like a team needs time to perform at its best, your body needs sufficient sleep to let its 'fighters' do their job. As the leader of your health, prioritize sleep to ensure your immune system operates at its best, reducing your risk of inflammatory disorders and other health issues.

Imagine this: after a busy week of late nights and early mornings, you finally reach the weekend feeling utterly exhausted. Then, just as you're hoping for some rest, you catch a cold that seems to stick around longer than usual.

What's happening behind the scenes? Your lack of sleep may have weakened your immune system, impairing its ability to fight off the virus effectively. This can result in extended inflammation and a prolonged recovery period. By allowing your body to rest and recuperate, you support your immune system's ability to handle inflammation and enhance your overall health in the long run.

So, how much sleep do you actually need? Although this will vary slightly from person to person, here is a list of how much sleep is required per night for different age groups:

- Newborns (0-3 months): 14-17 hours
- Infants (4-11 months): 12-15 hours
- Toddlers (1-2 years): 11-14 hours
- Preschoolers (3-5 years): 10-13 hours
- School-age children (6-13 years): 9-11 hours
- Teenagers (14-17 years): 8-10 hours
- Younger adults (18-25 years): 7-9 hours
- Adults (26-64 years): 7-9 hours
- Older adults (65 years and above): 7-8 hours

Crafting better sleep habits

So by now it's fairly obvious that sleep is crucial for our overall health, especially if you're trying to heal and fight things like infections and inflammation. But you're busy and have a lot going on, so how can you get a better night's sleep? Now that you have a better understanding of sleep, you've already implemented the first stages of your journey toward healing through food and exercise. These next steps will be like a walk in the park. Let's go through a few ways you can craft better habits for a more restful sleep.

1. Remove external distractions - Remove and turn off electronics from your sleep environment, especially cell phones, which omit high-frequency signals that can affect you while you sleep. Light from TV, clocks, or digital readouts can also affect your sleep pattern. Turning them off is best practice so they don't interfere with your sleep cycles.

2. Schedule and consistency - Go to bed at night and wake up in the morning at the same time every day. Consistency is key to creating habits and maintaining them. Sticking to a schedule also reinforces the natural sleep-wake cycle (circadian rhythm).

3. Food consciousness - Pay attention to what you eat, as food can directly influence your sleep patterns and schedule. Heavy meals, caffeine, and sugar will affect both your ability to fall asleep and the quality of sleep. Avoiding food a few hours before bed is recommended, remember we naturally fast at night, and trying to digest while we sleep interferes with our sleep patterns. (Refer back to Chapter 2 for information about healthy eating habits and fasting practices.)

4. Alcohol, tobacco, and recreational drugs - These habits can significantly impact your sleep quality and cycles. Alcohol might initially make you feel drowsy, but it disrupts your sleep stages, particularly REM sleep, leading to fragmented rest and reduced overall sleep quality. Tobacco, with its nicotine content, can interfere with your ability to fall asleep and maintain restful sleep, leading to increased wakefulness during the night. Recreational drugs, depending on their effects, can either make it difficult to fall asleep or lead to restless, non-refreshing sleep. To support healthy sleep patterns and overall well-being, it is crucial to avoid these substances or use them sparingly, focusing instead on healthy lifestyle choices that promote restorative sleep.

5. Limit and manage stress - Stress is the number one killer and can cause many sleepless and restless nights. Learn to manage your stress using methods and strategies from Chapter 4 to help you destress and sleep soundly. Don't let the worries from the day keep you awake!

6. Restful sleeping environment - Your sleeping space should be comfortable, dark, and semi-cool. A cooler temperature helps us to sleep better. For best sleep results your environment should be quiet, dark, cool, clean, and free from distractions.

7. Napping - Sleeping during the daytime can affect your natural sleep-wake cycle. Avoid napping regularly unless you are sick or injured or for other circumstances such as fatigue from travel or work.

8. Physical activity and nature - Especially when combined physical activity outdoors can help you sleep like a baby. Remember beach days when you were a kid, I bet like me you were passed out in the back of the old volts-wagon before you even got home. Move your body regularly and go outside for some fun. Both positively affect your whole self and will help your body and brain relax faster to fall asleep and sleep deeper for repair and recovery.

9. Know when to get help - Sleeplessness and insomnia can be a serious problem for many people, especially for those who have conditions such as restless legs, apnea, or other serious health issues. Consult a physician or professional to ensure you are not at risk of serious conditions or are already having symptoms as a result of something deeper going on. Know yourself, and when to ask for help!

Here are a few tips and strategies to help you fall asleep faster.

- **Listen to soothing music** or a white noise machine: These can help mask disruptive noises and create a calming atmosphere. Avoid falling asleep to TV noise, which can be stimulating and disruptive.

- **Try natural remedies**: Instead of medication, consider herbal tea, aromatherapy, or meditation (see the how-to guide below).

- Avoid blue light before bed: Blue light from TVs, phones, computers, and tablets can interfere with your sleep. Keep these devices out of your sleeping area.

- **Turn off Wi-Fi and data on phones**: These devices emit frequencies that can disrupt your sleep cycle. Keep phones away from the bed.

- **Recite positive affirmations**, recollect good memories, or express gratitude: This helps put you in a relaxed and happy state, making it easier to fall asleep.

- **Establish a bedtime routine**: Create a calming pre-sleep ritual, such as reading a book, taking a warm bath, or practicing gentle yoga.

- **Keep a consistent sleep schedule**: Go to bed and wake up at the same time every day, even on weekends, to regulate your internal clock.

- **Create a comfortable sleep environment**: Ensure your bedroom is cool, dark, and quiet. Invest in a comfortable mattress and pillows.

- **Limit caffeine and heavy meals**: Avoid consuming caffeine and large, heavy meals close to bedtime, as they can interfere with your ability to fall asleep.

- **Stay physically active**: Regular exercise can help you fall asleep faster and enjoy deeper sleep, but avoid vigorous activity close to bedtime.

How to Meditate Before You Sleep

Meditating before bed can help calm your mind and prepare your body for restful sleep. Here's a simple guide to get you started:

1. **Find a Quiet Space** - Choose a quiet, comfortable spot where you won't be disturbed. You can add this meditation also to your bedtime routine.

2. **Get Comfortable** - Sit or lie down in a relaxed position. Close your eyes and take a few deep breaths.

3. **Focus on Your Breathing** - Breathe deeply and slowly. Focus on the sensation of your breath entering and leaving your body.

4. **Visualize Calm** - Imagine a peaceful scene, like a beach or a forest. Focus on the details to immerse yourself in the tranquility.

5. **Body Scan** - Gradually bring your attention to each part of your body, starting from your toes and moving up to your head. Notice any tension and consciously relax those areas.

6. **Mantra or Affirmation** - Silently repeat a calming word or phrase, such as "relax" or "peace," to maintain focus.

7. **Let Go of Thoughts** - If your mind wanders, gently bring your focus back to your breath or your mantra. Don't judge the wandering; just guide your attention back.

8. **Gradual Return** - As your session ends, slowly become aware of your surroundings. Stretch gently and open your eyes. It's also okay if you fall asleep!

Tips for success:

- Consistency - Meditate at the same time each night to establish a routine.
- Environment - Dim the lights and reduce noise to create a soothing atmosphere.
- Patience - It might take some time to get used to meditation. Be patient and persistent.

By incorporating this meditation practice into your bedtime routine, you can enhance the quality of your sleep and wake up feeling refreshed.

Chapter checklist

Understanding your Sleep Patterns:

- ☐ Learn about the stages of sleep (N1, N2, N3, REM Sleep) and their significance in physical and mental recovery.
- ☐ Understand the importance of sleep in maintaining overall health and well-being, including its role in brain and body restoration.

Exploring the Role of Sleep and Inflammation:

- ☐ Recognize how sleep impacts the immune system and its ability to regulate inflammation.
- ☐ Explore studies and evidence linking poor sleep with increased levels of inflammation.
- ☐ Understand the potential health consequences of disrupted or insufficient sleep on inflammatory disorders and heart disease.

Improve your Sleep Habits:

- ☐ Discover practical tips for improving sleep quality and duration, including sticking to a consistent sleep schedule and creating a restful sleep environment.

☐ Learn about the importance of nutrition, physical activity, and stress management in promoting better sleep.

☐ Explore strategies for managing worries and limiting exposure to screens and caffeine before bedtime.

Learn how to keep a sleep diary to assess your sleep patterns.

Template Example

Date: [Insert Date]

Instructions:

- Fill out the sleep diary every morning upon waking up.
- Be as detailed and honest as possible in your responses.
- Use the diary to identify patterns and adjust your sleep habits for improved sleep quality.
- Refer to previous entries to track progress over time and make informed decisions about your sleep routine.

Prompts to use:

1. Describe your bedtime routine and any activities you engaged in before sleep.
2. What factors influenced the quality of your sleep environment (e.g., temperature, noise)?
3. How long did you sleep, and did you feel well-rested upon waking up?
4. Were there any interruptions or disturbances during your sleep?
5. How did you feel upon waking up, and did you notice any changes in your mood or energy levels throughout the day?
6. Did you take any naps during the day, and if so, how did they affect your overall sleep quality?
7. Reflect on any patterns or trends you observed in your sleep habits.
8. Is there anything you would like to change or improve about your sleep routine based on today's experience?

Use this sleep diary to track your sleep patterns and make adjustments to optimize your sleep quality and overall well-being.

With a deeper understanding of the science behind sleep and its impact on inflammation, it's time to take actionable steps toward crafting better sleep habits. By implementing changes to improve sleep quality and duration, you'll not only enhance your overall health but also reduce the risk of inflammatory disorders and promote a healthier, more balanced lifestyle.

Chapter 6 - C.A.L.M.N.**E**.S.S.

E - Enhance Lifestyle Choices

Remember when you sat down for that "grown-up talk" after coming home late from a party; you were told how the choices you make now will have a lasting impact on the rest of your life. How it's important to make good choices, respect your elders, and blah, blah, blah… Like me, you probably tuned out at this point. But you got the point: be nice, follow the rules, don't do drugs or alcohol, smoking is bad for your health, and so on. Okay, so I don't want you to think this chapter is another speech about lifestyle choices, so don't go having flashbacks about that awkward conversation you were forced to have. Instead, let this chapter be an educational discussion or at least a reminder of some important facts about healthy lifestyle choices you may have forgotten.

We are on this journey toward taming inflammation together, and I'd hate for you to skip through because you already "heard all this before." Just bear with me through this chapter as we cover how lifestyle choices really do impact our body, especially inflammation. So far you've made huge strides and changes, this chapter is just another step toward healing. Before we get into the facts let's take some inspiration from Jess, who's lifestyle changes have had a lasting and positive impact.

Jess had been struggling to lose weight and manage her chronic back pain for years. Inspired by a friend Jess decided to see a lifestyle coach for a consultation. After just one conversation, Jess understood that many of her everyday choices greatly impacted her health. Jess had already adopted a healthy diet, food in her case wasn't the issue. However, she enjoyed iced coffees, lattes, diet soda, and wine every night. Jess was also an occasional smoker and spent weekends sleeping and staying up late. Sure she walked on her lunch breaks and ate fairly well, yet all these other small habits and addictions were causing triggers and were counterproductive to her progress.

Jess can admit it wasn't easy, but right away she switched out her calorie-rich drinks to more water and herbal teas. Jess cut back on wine as well and started a program to help her kick cigarettes for good. And last she kept a more regular sleeping routine and incorporated chair exercises three times a week. At first, she didn't see any results but Jess was determined so she kept with it. By maintaining a more holistic lifestyle and becoming more conscious of the little things compromising her ability to heal, She was finally able to reach her goals. Jess started with small changes that led to a huge outcome for her; the little things make all the difference, and we are in charge. We get to choose how we live and when it is time to make changes.

To Drink or Not to Drink? How Alcohol Affects Your Body!

For many people and cultures around the world alcohol is a right of passage to adulthood. It's how we celebrate special occasions, how we remember people and it's often served in every gathering space, and in this day and age, it's around every corner. Alcohol is a normal part of many people's lives, however, it seems we have mistakenly put this product on such a pedestal when it brings so much darkness and as well learn better at physical health problems. That's not to say you shouldn't drink alcohol, however. Understanding what alcohol is, and how it affects us can help us make informed decisions about how we choose to live and heal.

Alcohol-Inflammation Connection

What is alcohol?

Alcohol is a substance found in beer, wine, and spirits, such as vodka, whiskey, and tequila. It is produced through the fermentation or distillation of sugars and grains.

How Alcohol Works:

- **Brain Impact** - Alcohol acts as a depressant, slowing down brain activity and responses. This can lead to feelings of relaxation, lowered inhibitions, impaired coordination, judgment, and reaction times.

- **Health Effects** - Moderate alcohol consumption might have some social benefits, but excessive drinking can lead to numerous health issues such as liver disease, heart problems, and increased risk of accidents. It can also contribute to mental health issues like depression and anxiety.

- **Addiction** - Alcohol can be highly addictive, and regular consumption can lead to dependence, requiring higher amounts to achieve the same effects and causing withdrawal symptoms when not consumed.

- **Calories and Nutritional Value** - Alcoholic beverages often contain a high number of calories with little to no nutritional value, which can contribute to weight gain and poor nutrition if consumed excessively.

- **Legal and Social Impact** - The legal drinking age varies by country, and alcohol consumption is often regulated. Socially, alcohol can play a significant role in cultural and social activities but can also lead to negative consequences like impaired driving and social conflicts when abused.

Can alcohol affect inflammation?

The short answer is: yes! But why? Well, that's the interesting part. Besides the obvious drunk feeling and behavior issues on the outside, on the inside alcohol is wreaking havoc and fueling fire everywhere it goes.

As soon as your body begins to digest alcohol it begins to produce inflammatory compounds as it gets broken down. The alcohol leaves behind by-products that damage your gut, liver, and other organs.

According to a 2023 study done by The International Journal of Molecular Science, Acetaldehyde is a harmful toxin produced from the alcohol metabolism process. Although Acetaldehyde is short-lived in our bodies it causes serious damage to major organs like the liver, brain, and pancreas. This toxin along with others like cytokines, chemo lines, and reactive oxygen species (ROS) all insight an inflammatory response.

Alcohol is the catalyst for inflammation, as the toxins cause oxidative stress and cell damage. Alcohol disrupts all our essential mechanisms and our overall defensive system (AKA: Immune system). Alcohol increases the permeability in your intestines, allowing more bacteria and toxins to leak into your bloodstream, disrupting healthy bacteria and causing an inflammatory response. Over time this can cause systemic (body-wide) inflammation, which can lead to gastrointestinal, autoimmune, cardiovascular, metabolic, and neurological diseases.

Oxidative stress from alcohol can result in an imbalance between the free radicals and antioxidants in your body leading to confusion, fueling inflammation, and possibly laying the path for heart disease, respiratory disorders, and even cancer. This stress on your body and organs also puts you at a greater risk for inflammatory diseases, obesity, and diabetes. Alcohol has serious health consequences and should be avoided when possible. Moderation is key if you plan to consume or abstain completely, and this is all without even mentioning the calories in some of the most popular drinks. Yikes! That could be an entire chapter on its own.

The Broad Impact of Smoking

It's no secret tobacco and secondhand smoke are deadly, but to what degree does it affect our health, specifically our inflammation? Let's dive deep into the effects of smoking so we can better understand how this lifestyle choice could impact your healing journey.

The fact is that in just America alone over 16 million people are living with a smoke-related disease which leads to premature death for 6 million people worldwide. These statistics alone are scary enough but let's dive deeper. What does smoking do to you?

Smoking harms nearly every organ and cell in the body, causing numerous diseases and reducing overall health. It increases the risk of various cancers, including lung, throat, and cervical cancer, and contributes significantly to heart disease, leading to higher chances of heart attacks and strokes. Smoking also leads to chronic obstructive pulmonary diseases like emphysema and chronic bronchitis and raises the risk of developing type 2 diabetes. Furthermore, it disrupts immune function and elevates white blood cell levels, resulting in increased inflammation. Other health impacts include a higher likelihood of developing tuberculosis, eye diseases, and rheumatoid arthritis.

Secondhand smoke poses additional risks, causing coronary heart disease, stroke, and lung cancer in non-smokers. For children, exposure to secondhand smoke increases the risk of sudden infant death syndrome (SIDS), acute respiratory infections, middle ear disease, severe asthma, and other respiratory symptoms, while also slowing their growth.

Smoking also depletes nutrients, lowering the effectiveness of antioxidants like vitamin C and reducing bone density. It adversely affects reproductive health by decreasing sperm count and increasing sperm deformities in men, while lowering fertility, disrupting menstrual cycles, and raising the risk of cervical cancer in women. Digestive health is compromised with a higher risk of stomach and intestinal inflammation and ulcers. Additionally, smoking increases the risk of blindness, leads to premature wrinkles, causes gum disease, and ultimately increases the risk of early death.

There's no way to make any of that sound good—it's horrible! But these are the facts of what happens when you smoke or are exposed to secondhand smoke. All of these side effects weaken essential processes in our bodies, such as our immune system, making it harder to fight off diseases, viruses, and bacteria. Additionally, smoking fuels inflammation, exacerbating chronic conditions. Overall, smoking is one of the worst lifestyle choices we can make, especially when dealing with inflammation.

Supporting the Immune System

We've discussed the immune system several times already. Maintaining a healthy immune system involves a balanced diet, regular exercise, staying hydrated, getting enough sleep, managing stress, and practicing good hygiene. Avoiding alcohol and tobacco also supports immune health. However, there are additional ways to boost immunity, especially during cold and flu season or at the onset of illness.

Incorporating superfoods like berries, leafy greens, and legumes into your diet can significantly enhance your immune function. These foods are rich in antioxidants and micronutrients vital for a robust immune system. If you find it challenging to consume a diverse variety of foods, supplements can help, but they should only be used if advised by a healthcare professional.

Consider getting regular check-ups with your physician to ensure your immune system is working correctly. Early detection is the best way to ensure you get proper treatment before issues persist or turn into chronic conditions. Regular checkups are a great habit to get into for the whole family.

Here is a list of screening tests that the entire family should have done regularly as a preventative measure.

<ins>Annual wellness checkups</ins>

- o Blood pressure
- o Body mass index (BMI)
- o Dental exams
- o Physical exam
- o Preventive screening
- o Counseling

Recommended Cancer screenings

- Colorectal
- Skin
- Breast (women)
- Cervical (women)
- Testicular and Prostate (men)

Sensory screenings

- Eyesight
- Hearing (only if symptoms arise)

Immunizations: Staying Up to Date

Vaccinations are essential for maintaining a strong immune system and protecting against various diseases. However, it's important to note that some vaccines have a limited period of effectiveness and require periodic renewals to ensure continued protection. Here is a recommended schedule for common vaccinations:

- **Tetanus, Diphtheria (Tdap):** A booster shot every 10 years. If you haven't had Tdap before, it's recommended to get one dose, followed by Td booster shots every 10 years.
- **Influenza:** Annually, typically in the fall.
- **Pneumococcal:** Once after age 65 or as recommended by your healthcare provider.
- **MMR (Measles, Mumps, Rubella):** Two doses in childhood; a booster may be needed for some adults.
- **Meningococcal:** Every 5 years if at continued risk.
- Varicella (Chickenpox): Two doses if not previously immunized.
- **Shingles:** One dose after age 50.
- **Human Papillomavirus (HPV):** Two to three doses depending on age at first vaccination.
- **Hepatitis A:** Two doses, six months apart.
- **Hepatitis B:** Three doses over six months.
- Haemophilus Influenzae Type B (Hib): Usually given in

childhood, but may be recommended for certain adults.

For a detailed and personalized vaccination schedule, refer to the CDC's Adult Immunization Schedule (CDC). This page provides the latest recommendations and helps ensure you stay up-to-date with your vaccinations.

Keeping up with vaccinations is critical to maintaining a strong immune system and overall health. Consult your healthcare provider to tailor the schedule to your specific needs.

Practicing Self-Care

I used to think self-care was just for grandmas and posh people, but it turns out that every single person should be practicing self-care! Especially for those of us who work hard every day, taking care of yourself should be a top priority.

Self-care can be as simple or as luxurious as you want. It involves activities that care for your body and mind, helping you relax, cleanse, or escape from the stresses life puts on you physically, emotionally, and mentally. Self-care can be as simple as hydrating your skin with lotion or taking a bath after a day spent under dry lights and air conditioning, or as luxurious as a week-long spa vacation being pampered from head to toe.

Taking time for self-care is not just a luxury; it's essential. It has been clinically proven to reduce or eliminate anxiety and depression, lower stress, increase happiness, improve concentration, minimize anger and frustration, boost energy, and reduce the risk of heart disease and stroke.

Like stress management practices, self-care can have a ricochet of benefits. Self-care isn't just herbal baths and yoga. We can practice self-care in every aspect of our lives to create an ongoing habit that will help make life easier. However, keep in mind we are all individuals, and self-care practices, and results will differ from person to person.

Emotional care: Don't be afraid to talk to someone, reflect, and journal about emotional troubles, worries, and stresses. Escape into a good book, some good music, or a feel-good or funny movie. Eat healthy food, exercise, go for a walk, get artsy or creative. Cry it out if you need to, hug somebody you love, and don't ignore your emotions.

Spiritual care: Meditation, prayer, and reflection have many benefits including helping you to find clarity in your life's purpose, and it can help you connect to your inner power. These practices also can lead to better responses to frustrating situations, build better relationships, and solve problems more easily.

Physical care: Healthy food and regular workouts are top priorities for your body. But, don't forget to get regular checkups at the doctor and dentist, and move without a routine like nature walks, summer swims, and fun physical activities. Most importantly avoid drugs, alcohol, and tobacco.

Intellectual care: Our brains are muscles and we must work them out as well, especially for self-care incorporating things like reading, listening to audiobooks, watching informative documentaries, crafting puzzles, being curious and asking questions, trying something new, being creative, and learning new skills. These are all activities to enhance your brain and emotions, not to mention give you more fulfillment and purpose, as you grow your wealth of knowledge and experience.

Social care: in this day and age, we are more connected than ever and it's important to remember our social self-care practices will help us regulate our stress while maximizing 'caring for yourself'. Staying in contact and meeting up with friends and family who don't bring negativity to you or others. Make time to go out and have fun with friends or family, watch positive content and people. Try volunteering, being kind and giving your services and experience, living life through love, and most importantly ignoring negative people and comments.

More self-care tips:

1. **Call or Text Someone You Love** - Connecting with loved ones can boost your mood and reduce stress.

2. **Drink a Cup of Tea or Coffee** - Enjoying a warm beverage can be soothing and comforting.

3. **Journal About How You're Feeling** - Writing down your thoughts helps process emotions and relieve stress.

4. **Take Deep Breaths** - Practicing deep breathing can reduce anxiety and promote relaxation.

5. **Listen to Your Favorite Music** - Music can be uplifting and help you feel more positive.

6. **Go for a Long Walk in Nature** - Being in nature can enhance your mood and provide a sense of peace.

7. **Cook or Order Your Favorite Meal** - Enjoying a favorite dish can be a comforting and satisfying experience.

8. **Read a Book** - Escaping into a book can provide a mental break and help you relax.

9. **Light Your Favorite Candle** - The soothing scents of a candle can create a calming atmosphere.

10. **Do a Digital Detox** - Taking a break from screens can help you reset and focus on the present.

11. **Go to Your Favorite Place** - Visiting a place you love can bring comfort and joy.

12. **Stretch** - Stretching can relieve physical tension and improve your overall well-being.

13. **Try a New Face Mask** - Pampering your skin can be a relaxing and refreshing activity.

14. **Read Inspirational Quotes** - Positive quotes can inspire and uplift your spirits.

15. **Get Some Sleep** - Prioritizing rest can significantly improve your mood and energy levels.

16. **Organize or Rearrange Your Space** - A tidy space can lead to a tidy mind, reducing stress.

17. **Buy Yourself Flowers** - Treating yourself to something beautiful can brighten your day.

18. **Exercise in a Way That Feels Good for You** - Physical activity can boost your mood and health.

19. **Write Down 5 Things You're Grateful For** - Practicing gratitude can enhance your overall well-being.

20. **Spend Quality Time with Friends or Family** - Spend time with people who are supportive, encouraging, and have a positive impact on you. Try also spending time with pets or other animals, they can have a positive effect on your mental health. Social connections are vital for emotional support and happiness.

Cultivate Positive Thinking

Our bodies and minds are not disconnected. They work together to maintain a healthy environment. Scientific studies show us that hormones and neurotransmitters or chemical messengers associated with emotions can have physical effects and they can affect your blood pressure, heart rate, and even your appetite. Remember when we discussed stress in Chapter 4 and the hormones that kick in the fight or flight response? Those are the same hormones released during an emotional state; as you know, those hormones directly impact our immune system and overall mechanisms for maintaining health.

Imagine this: You've spent the last couple of weeks meticulously planning a summer family picnic, excited to reunite everyone after years of being too busy. However, two nights before the event, you begin to worry about all sorts of scenarios—food poisoning grandma, cousins Billy and John getting into a fight, or the dog eating all the food. These thoughts keep you awake, and the day before the picnic, you lose your appetite and avoid eating altogether. Despite your fears, everyone arrives on time, the day is a success, and plans for next year's picnic are already in the works.

Now, consider how different things might have been if you had been able to manage your stress effectively. If you had been able to relax, eat well, and get enough sleep before the gathering, your immune system would have been in better shape, potentially preventing any stress-related symptoms. Healthy eating and adequate sleep are crucial for maintaining a strong immune system, which is better equipped to handle the emotional stress and worry that can impact your well-being. Emotional worry and fear directly affect your immune system, and managing these stressors through positive reinforcement and self-care can make a significant difference in your overall health.

It's easy to understand that emotions and stress, which release hormones, can impact your physical health, but what about the power of your thoughts? Would you believe it if I told you that what you think can also affect your physical and overall health? Studies have shown that negative thinking can trigger stress hormones, fueling the fire of inflammation. Your thoughts play a significant role in your healing journey, either positively or negatively. Adopting positive thinking habits can serve as another tool in your arsenal against illness and inflammation.

This doesn't mean that becoming more optimistic will prevent you from responding appropriately to sadness or anger. However, practicing mindfulness and positive thinking will make coping with stress and hardships easier. Embracing a positive mindset can help mitigate the harmful effects of stress hormones, aiding in your overall well-being and reducing inflammation in the body.

Benefits of becoming more optimistic and positive:

- Increased life span
- Lowers rates of depression, distress, and pain
- Greater resistance to illness
- Better, psychological and physical
- Better cardiovascular health and lower risk of heart disease

and stroke
- Reduce risk of death by cancer respiratory conditions in infection
- Better coping skills

Staying positive can significantly expand your awareness and make you more open to new ideas, fostering personal growth. This mindset allows you to see opportunities and solutions that might otherwise be overlooked when consumed by negativity. By embracing positivity, you become more receptive to learning and adapting, which can lead to greater resilience and an enhanced ability to handle life's challenges. This openness not only supports your mental well-being but also contributes to your overall personal development.

Strategies to try:

As an optimist, it's important to...

- **Give yourself credit for good deeds** - Reflect every day on the good you have done, the nice things you said, etc.

- **Forgive yourself** - Everyone makes mistakes. What did you or can you learn from it? Every mistake is a lesson to learn from.

- **Spend time with positive friends and family** - People who are encouraging, and supportive talk about the future in a positive way. Of course, you also reciprocate support and love. And, don't be afraid to remove toxic, negative people or relationships to better your healing journey.

- **Explore your meaning of life** - What principles do you live by and how can that guide you to live to your potential to find or make purpose?

- **Develop healthy lifestyle habits** - Following all the stages within these chapters. Healthy eating. Physical activity. Proper sleep habits, mindfulness, and thinking more positively.

More ways to stay positive...

- Focus on the good things

- Practice gratitude every day

- Keep a gratitude journal (it's all about the little things)

- Open yourself up to humor, smile, and laugh more.

- Practice positive self-talk, " I've got this, I will try again, I've learned, I can make it happen, I did a good job, I am enough!"

- Identify your areas of negativity: these may be habits, thought processes, relationships, or situations, and consciously be aware and remove yourself or make changes and new habits.

- Start every day on a positive note, avoid the news, conflict, and negative energy, listen to music, exercise, listen to the birds, etc.

You got this!

Chapter checklist

Let's think about your own situation based on the chapter topics. Don't forget to take notes and jot down your thoughts and observations as you go through the checklist.

To drink or not to drink alcohol?

☐ Understand how alcohol contributes to inflammation.

☐ Learn moderation techniques and explore healthier alternatives to reduce its inflammatory effects.

Understand the Impact of Smoking on Inflammation:

☐ Recognize the wide-ranging health consequences of smoking.

☐ Learn about the direct link between smoking and increased inflammatory markers.

☐ Understand the effects of vaping on inflammation.

Implement Lifestyle Changes to boost your Immune System:

- ☐ Explore strategies to strengthen your immune system, such as a balanced diet, regular exercise, and stress management.
- ☐ Emphasize the importance of regular health check-ups and monitoring.
- ☐ List common health check-ups to ensure proactive health management.

Integrate Self-Care Practices into Daily Your Routines:

- ☐ Understand the importance of self-care for mental and physical health.
- ☐ Discover practical self-care ideas to incorporate into your life for stress reduction and well-being.

Practice Positive Thinking to Support Your Physical Health:

- ☐ Learn the science behind the mind-body connection.
- ☐ Understand how positive thinking can influence physical health.
- ☐ Explore strategies to develop a more optimistic outlook, such as practicing gratitude and positive self-talk.

Self-Care Tracker

To help you incorporate self-care into your daily routine, use this interactive self-care tracker that includes journal prompts, a happiness checklist, and a self-care to-do list. This will help you stay mindful of your self-care practices and track your progress.

Daily Journal Prompts

- Morning Reflection: What am I grateful for today?
- Midday Check-in: How am I feeling right now?
- What can I do to improve my mood?
- Evening Reflection: What was the best part of my day?
- Self-Care Evaluation: Did I make time for self-care today?
- How did it make me feel?

Happiness Checklist

- Did I laugh or smile today?
- Did I take a moment to appreciate something beautiful?
- Did I engage in a hobby or activity that I love?
- Did I spend time with friends or family?
- Did I practice mindfulness or meditation?
- Did I exercise or move my body?

Self-Care To-Do List

- Drink at least 8 glasses of water.
- Get 7-9 hours of sleep.
- Eat a balanced meal.
- Spend at least 30 minutes doing something I enjoy.
- Take a short walk outside.
- Practice deep breathing or meditation for 5-10 minutes.
- Limit screen time, especially before bed.
- Write down three things I'm grateful for.

Weekly Review

1. **Achievements**: What self-care activities did I complete this week?
2. **Challenges**: What self-care activities did I find difficult to complete? Why?
3. **Goals**: What are my self-care goals for next week?
4. **Feelings**: How do I feel about my self-care practices this week?

Using the Tracker

- Daily Use: Spend a few minutes each day filling out the journal prompts and checking off items on your happiness checklist and self-care to-do list.
- Weekly Review: At the end of each week, reflect on your self-care practices and set goals for the upcoming week.

By consistently using this self-care tracker, you'll be able to nurture your well-being and make self-care an integral part of your lifestyle.

Having explored the various lifestyle adjustments that can help combat inflammation, it's time to broaden our perspective and turn to the natural world. In the next chapter, we will delve into how nature's bounty—through herbs, supplements, and other natural remedies—provides a wealth of anti-inflammatory benefits. From ancient herbal practices to modern scientific discoveries, we will uncover the potent power of natural elements in promoting health and reducing inflammation. Prepare to discover how integrating these natural remedies can further enhance your journey toward optimal well-being.

Chapter 7 - C.A.L.M.N.E.**S**.S.

S - Seek Natural Remedies and Knock on Nature's Pharmacy

"Nature itself is the best medicine."

Hippocrates

As you may have already noticed, the common theme throughout this book is that your healing journey is holistic and that nature itself is truly the best medicine. We thrive when we eat the healthiest whole foods grown from the earth. We feel amazing when we spend time outside doing physical activities, finding solace in simply listening to the sounds of nature around us. Nature is healing and an integral part of your journey to wellness. Let's delve deeper into the power of nature by understanding how to use herbs and simple natural remedies to support your healing process.

Ancient remedies and herbal cures have been used for centuries, yet they have recently been largely forgotten. It's time we reclaim this knowledge to reconnect with the earth that provides everything we need to achieve our health goals and live pain-free. Cultures worldwide have used herbs for healing, treatment, and prevention. Let's explore some easily accessible herbs, plants, and foods with healing properties that can help you combat inflammation.

Plants and herbs play a huge role in our healing process because many of these foods and plants have not only macronutrients and micronutrients but are full of compounds that work naturally with our bodies to help us heal, fight off infection, and prevent illness. Nature truly is amazing!

Most of these compounds we can get through a natural diet, however, there are times in certain individuals when supplements are required. Of course, speak to a healthcare provider before supplementing anything. Below is a list of some natural food sources that contain many healing compounds to help you fight against inflammation.

Garlic, one of my favorite ingredients! Garlic is rich in sulfur compounds like allicin, which have anti-inflammatory and immune-boosting effects. It helps reduce the risk of heart disease and has antibacterial properties. Garlic is so versatile, easy to grow, and relatively easy and cheap to find anywhere. Use fresh garlic in cooking, salads, sauces and so much more. Garlic supplements are also available. Beware, however, high doses might cause bad breath and digestive upset.

Ginseng has anti-inflammatory and antioxidant effects, which can help reduce oxidative stress and support immune function. You can add ginseng root to teas, soups, or smoothies. Ginseng supplements are also available. Be aware it might interact with medications, and cause side effects like insomnia or digestive issues in high doses.

Cardamom also has anti-inflammatory and antioxidant properties, which can help reduce blood pressure and improve digestive health. Cardamom is common in East Asia and is a dish, but you'll find it used around the world in teas, desserts, and more. Try enjoying a chai tea made with cardamom and other beneficial anti-inflammatory herbs such as black pepper, cinnamon, turmeric, and ginger.

Beware: cardamom and other spices are generally safe, but high doses may cause mild allergic reactions. Too much cinnamon, especially cassia cinnamon, can lead to liver toxicity due to high levels of coumarin. Always consume any foods, herbs, or supplements in moderation, a little goes a long way.

Try these anti-inflammatory chai tea recipes!

Golden Turmeric Chai

Ingredients:

- 1 cup almond milk (or milk of choice)
- 1 cup water
- 1 black tea bag
- 1 tsp turmeric powder
- 1/2 tsp ground cinnamon
- 1/2 tsp ground ginger
- 1/4 tsp ground cardamom
- 1/4 tsp ground black pepper
- 1 tbsp honey or maple syrup (optional)

Instructions:

1. In a saucepan, combine almond milk and water and bring to a gentle boil.
2. Add the black tea bag and steep for 3-5 minutes.
3. Remove the tea bag and stir in turmeric, cinnamon, ginger, cardamom, and black pepper.
4. Reduce heat and simmer for 5 minutes.
5. Strain the tea into a mug and sweeten with honey or maple syrup if desired. Enjoy warm.

Ginger Cinnamon Chai

Ingredients:

- 2 cups water
- 1 black tea bag
- 1-inch piece of fresh ginger, sliced

- 1 cinnamon stick
- 2-3 whole cloves
- 1/4 tsp ground cardamom
- 1 cup coconut milk (or milk of choice)
- 1 tbsp honey or agave syrup (optional)

Instructions:

1. In a saucepan, bring water to a boil.
2. Add the black tea bag, ginger slices, cinnamon stick, cloves, and ground cardamom. Simmer for 10 minutes.
3. Add coconut milk and simmer for another 5 minutes.
4. Strain the tea into a mug.
5. Sweeten with honey or agave syrup if desired. Serve hot.

Ginger, although delicious in tea, is also good in many dishes, both sweet and savory. Like ginger and roaster carrot soup, or ginger and garlic veggies spring rolls...yum! Ginger contains gingerol, a bioactive compound with powerful anti-inflammatory and antioxidant properties. It can help reduce muscle pain and soreness, as well as symptoms of osteoarthritis. On a side note, excessive consumption may cause digestive issues, moderation is key.

Green Tea, another one of my favorites! whether you are a fan or not Green tea is rich in polyphenols, particularly epigallocatechin gallate (EGCG), which have strong anti-inflammatory and antioxidant properties. It's tea, drink it hot or cold at least three times a day or use green tea extract in smoothies and other recipes. Beware excessive consumption can lead to caffeine-related side effects such as insomnia and increased heart rate.

Rosemary, another delicious and beneficial herb. (Our spice racks are looking more like medicine cabinets, wouldn't you agree?) Rosemary contains carnosic acid and rosmarinic acid, which have anti-inflammatory effects and can improve digestion and brain function. Use fresh or dried rosemary in cooking, such as in soups, stews, and roasted meats. Of course, be aware large amounts might cause stomach upset or allergic reactions in some people.

Turmeric is used worldwide for its color, its flavor, and its medicinal properties! Turmeric contains curcumin, a potent anti-inflammatory compound that can help with arthritis and reduce inflammation markers. Turmeric can be used to flavor curries, soups, dressing, smoothies, and more. Combine with black pepper to enhance absorption. Try the tea recipes from above. Be aware that excessive intake may cause digestive issues and interact with certain medications.

Black Pepper: The Piperine in black pepper enhances the absorption of curcumin and other nutrients and has anti-inflammatory effects on its own. Pepper is common in almost every kitchen so this ingredient isn't hard to use. When it's time to season vegetables or proteins, remember a little extra pepper can go a long way. If you're not a fan of pepper you can add it to sauces, dressing, and marinades to help it blend in with other flavors.

There are so many plants that have medicinal properties. This list focuses on the plants with the highest compounds to help fight inflammation. Many herbs, flowers, and other garden plants can also be used medicinally to help boost the immune system, fight off infection, and give you extra vitamins,amins, and so forth.

Using herbs and these healing foods in your diet is just another tool in your arsenal toward taming inflammation for good; And, if you're interested in healing through plants, I encourage you to learn more about herbalism, Chinese medicine, or learning more about plants that are in your backyard. You'll find healing compounds in many weeds, garden plants, and roots that grow in your area. I encourage you to learn more if this interests you and if you're interested in learning about growing, let's move on to the next section, and get some quick tips on how to start a medicine garden at home.

Creating a medicinal garden is a rewarding activity that provides fresh, therapeutic herbs at your fingertips. Selecting the right plants is crucial, especially those with known health benefits that you'll actually use. Here's how to get started with some beginner-friendly choices, including anti-inflammatory plants.

Choosing the Right Plants for You

When starting a medicinal garden, it's important to choose plants known for their therapeutic properties and suitable for your local climate. Here are some great options for beginners:

- **Aloe Vera**: Renowned for its soothing gel, aloe vera is perfect for minor cuts and burns.

- **Lavender**: With its calming effects, lavender can be used in teas, sachets, and essential oils.

- **Mint**: This versatile herb aids digestion and can be used in teas, salads, and as a garnish.

- **Echinacea**: Known for its immune-boosting properties, echinacea is often used in teas and supplements.

- **Chamomile**: Famous for its relaxing qualities, chamomile can help with sleep and digestion.

Don't forget to incorporate anti-inflammatory plants like turmeric, ginger, garlic, and rosemary, provided your climate allows for their growth.

Choosing a Location

Sunlight: Most medicinal herbs require at least six hours of direct sunlight daily. When selecting a location, whether it's a sunny windowsill indoors or a spot in your garden, ensure your herbs will receive ample light.

Accessibility: Place your garden near your kitchen or living space for convenience. Easy access encourages regular use of your herbs in daily cooking and home remedies.

Pots or Beds: Which to Use?

Pots: If you have limited space, pots are an excellent choice. They allow you to control the soil quality and move plants as needed. Make sure the pots have good drainage to prevent waterlogging.

Raised Beds: For those with more space, raised beds are ideal. They offer better control over soil conditions and drainage. Ensure the soil is rich and well-draining to support healthy plant growth.

Tips for Care and Maintenance

Soil: Use well-draining soil enriched with organic matter, as it retains moisture while allowing excess water to drain away, thereby preventing root rot.

Watering: Regular watering is essential, but avoid overwatering. Most herbs prefer slightly moist soil but don't tolerate standing water.

Fertilizing: Use organic fertilizers sparingly. Over-fertilization can lead to excessive growth with less concentrated therapeutic properties.

Pest Control: Opt for natural pest control methods. Neem oil, for example, is effective against many pests without harming beneficial insects. Introducing beneficial insects like ladybugs can also help keep harmful pests in check.

Tips for Transplanting

Timing: Transplant seedlings in early spring after the last frost. This gives them the best chance to establish before the growing season.

Method: When transplanting, gently remove plants from their starter pots, taking care to loosen the roots. Plant them in their new location, ensuring the root ball is well-covered with soil. Water immediately to help them settle.

Tips for Harvesting

Timing: The best time to harvest herbs is in the morning, after the dew has dried, but before the sun is too strong. This is when the essential oils are most concentrated.

Method: Use sharp scissors or pruning shears to cut herbs above a leaf node. This encourages new growth and ensures a continuous supply of fresh herbs.

Creating a medicinal garden involves selecting the right plants, providing proper care, and using thoughtful harvesting techniques. Whether you're using pots or raised beds, a well-planned garden can offer a bountiful supply of therapeutic herbs to support your health and well-being.

Supplements for inflammation

Supplements can be a valuable addition to your health regimen, providing essential nutrients and compounds that may be lacking in your diet. They are particularly beneficial for reducing inflammation and supporting overall well-being. However, it's important to use them wisely and understand their benefits, proper dosages, and potential interactions with other medications or conditions. It's best practice to never start supplements without a consultation or recommendation from a doctor, health practitioner, or dietitian/nutritionist.

Bromelain: Found in the juicy core of pineapples, bromelain is a powerful enzyme known for its anti-inflammatory and digestive benefits. It can be particularly effective in reducing swelling and aiding in digestion. For those seeking its benefits in supplement form, a daily intake of 200-2,000 mg, divided into several doses, is common.

Cat's Claw: This vine, native to the Amazon rainforest, is celebrated for its immune-boosting and anti-inflammatory properties. While not typically found in everyday foods, cat's claw can be enjoyed as a tea or in supplement form, with a recommended dosage of 250-350 mg per day. Its unique compounds help in combating inflammation and supporting the immune system.

Curcumin (Turmeric): Curcumin, the active ingredient in turmeric, is a superstar in the world of anti-inflammatory agents. Known for its powerful antioxidant properties, curcumin is best absorbed with black pepper or fat. Daily supplementation ranges from 500-1,000 mg. Incorporate turmeric into your diet through curries, golden milk, or turmeric tea to harness its benefits.

Frankincense: Derived from the resin of the Boswellia tree, frankincense has been used for centuries to support joint health and reduce inflammation. Typically found as an essential oil or supplement, a common dosage is 300-400 mg of Boswellia extract taken 2-3 times a day. This ancient remedy can be particularly helpful for those with chronic inflammatory conditions.

Omega-3 Fatty Acids: Essential for reducing inflammation and supporting heart and brain health, omega-3 fatty acids are abundant in fatty fish, like salmon and mackerel, as well as in flaxseeds, chia seeds, and walnuts. Supplementation typically ranges from 1-3 grams per day, ensuring you receive these vital nutrients even if dietary sources are limited.

Quercetin: This flavonoid, found in apples, onions, and berries, boasts significant anti-inflammatory and antioxidant properties. To harness its benefits, a daily supplement dose of 500-1,000 mg is recommended. Adding more quercetin-rich foods to your diet can enhance your body's defense against inflammation.

Resveratrol: Resveratrol, famous for its presence in red wine and grapes, supports heart health and combats inflammation. With a typical supplement dosage of 150-500 mg per day, this compound helps protect the body against various inflammatory conditions.

Enjoying a moderate amount of red wine or snacking on grapes and berries can naturally boost your intake.

Spirulina: A nutrient-dense blue-green algae, spirulina is packed with antioxidants and anti-inflammatory properties. It can be added to smoothies or juices or taken as a supplement, with 1-3 grams per day being the common dosage. This superfood helps to bolster the body's defenses and improve overall health.

Vitamin D: Essential for immune function and reducing inflammation, vitamin D can be obtained from sunlight exposure, fatty fish, and fortified dairy products. Supplements, typically dosed at 1,000-2,000 IU per day, ensure adequate levels, especially in regions with limited sunlight.

Integrating these natural supplements and foods into your diet can significantly enhance your body's ability to fight inflammation and promote overall well-being. Whether through diet or supplementation, the power of nature's remedies is at your fingertips, ready to support a healthier, more balanced life.

Disclaimer

Before starting any new supplement, consult with a medical professional to ensure it's safe and appropriate for your individual health needs. Supplements should not replace a balanced diet or prescribed treatments and should be used as part of a comprehensive approach to health and wellness. Always follow the recommended dosage.

Other natural & Holistic treatments

Natural remedies can play a significant role in reducing inflammation and promoting overall wellness. Here are several methods, including their benefits and guidance on how to get started.

Acupuncture: Precise Healing with Ancient Techniques

Acupuncture, an ancient practice, involves inserting thin needles into specific points on the body to stimulate healing and pain relief. It is particularly effective for reducing chronic pain and inflammation, with some research indicating benefits for headaches, osteoarthritis, and other inflammatory conditions. When selecting an acupuncturist, ensure they have proper credentials and training. Look for reviews and referrals from trusted sources, and verify that they follow strict hygiene and safety standards to protect both you and them.

Massage Therapy: Healing Through Touch

Massage therapy is a hands-on technique that manipulates the body's soft tissues to relieve tension and pain. It's recommended to seek a licensed professional such as a physiotherapist, chiropractor, or massage therapist. Regular massage sessions can alleviate muscle pain and soreness, reduce stress, improve circulation, and promote relaxation. Different techniques are available, including Swedish massage for general relaxation and deep tissue massage for chronic muscle issues. Each method offers unique benefits, making massage therapy a versatile and effective treatment option for various conditions.

Hydrotherapy: Harnessing the Power of Water

Hydrotherapy, an age-old practice, uses water in its various forms—steam, ice, and liquid—to alleviate pain and treat numerous health conditions. The benefits of hydrotherapy are profound: it reduces muscle tension, eases pain, and enhances circulation, which in turn promotes healing. Starting with hydrotherapy can be as simple as taking warm baths infused with Epsom salts, providing significant relief. As you become more comfortable, you can explore advanced techniques like contrast baths, which involve alternating between hot and cold water to further enhance circulation and pain relief.

Aromatherapy: Healing Through Scent

Aromatherapy taps into the healing properties of essential oils derived from plants, offering a natural way to improve health and well-being. This practice is known to reduce anxiety, depression, and inflammation while also boosting mood and relaxation. To begin, you can use essential oils in diffusers to fill your space with therapeutic scents or add a few drops to your bath. Applying diluted oils topically can provide targeted relief for specific ailments, making aromatherapy a versatile tool in your wellness arsenal.

Cryotherapy: Embracing the Cold for Healing

Cryotherapy involves exposing the body to extremely cold temperatures, aiming to reduce inflammation and pain. This modern treatment can alleviate muscle pain, speed up recovery, boost immune function, and reduce chronic pain. Beginners should start with short sessions to allow the body to acclimate to the cold. It's crucial to wear appropriate clothing to protect sensitive areas during treatment. Cryotherapy sessions can be a brisk yet refreshing addition to your routine, providing a cold blast of therapeutic benefits.

Biofeedback: Mastering Your Body's Signals

Biofeedback is a fascinating technique that helps individuals learn to control physiological functions using real-time feedback from monitoring devices. These devices can track heart rate, muscle activity, skin temperature, and brain wave patterns. Biofeedback is typically conducted with a trained professional who can guide you through the process and help interpret the data. The benefits are substantial, including reduced stress, decreased muscle tension, and improved management of chronic pain and headaches. A typical biofeedback session involves attaching sensors to your body and learning techniques to modify bodily functions such as heart rate and muscle tension, empowering you to take control of your health in a new way.

Connecting with Nature

Nature has transformative and healing powers and comes in so many forms; food, fresh air, grounding, medicine, water, and of course, beauty. It's like nature was somehow created or left here just for us, kind of amazing!

Embracing nature inside and spending more time outside has so many benefits. These benefits include:

- Lowering stress
- Reduce social isolation
- Builds confidence
- Improves focus
- Reduces risk of depression
- Increases motivation to exercise
- Improves relaxation

Eco therapy can be part of your healing journey. This activity and therapy can be done individually or with a group and guided by an expert. Eco therapy takes place in a natural environment surrounded by greenery. Ecotherapy is based on one activity done in a natural setting to help remove focus from your internal self and focus on the healing powers of aiming and being active outside. An outdoor therapy session might involve exploring a specific location, such as a brook at the edge of a forest or a cluster of trees. By immersing yourself in the natural environment, you become more aware of the sounds, smells, and sights around you. This experience can be meditative, promoting both physical and mental well-being.

Ways to expose yourself to more nature

There are lots of ways to connect to nature, whether that's true Eco therapy, eating Whole Foods, planting a medicinal garden, or just spending more time outside. Here are some tips for connecting with nature, and bringing more nature into your life every day.

- Bring plants inside
- Add a water feature indoors
- Take breaks outside
- Walk and or exercise outside
- Try gardening
- Visit nature, sites, parks, and natural wonders
- Learn a new outdoor hobby, (hiking, skiing, canoeing, fishing, etc)
- Plan a nature trip

Imagine this: It's been a long week, physically and mentally you are exhausted and worst off your legs and feet are inflamed and you just want to get off of them for as long as possible. Unfortunately, life goes on, you still have to get up to pee, make coffee, walk the dog, and so forth. However, by now you are armed with the knowledge to take charge of your healing journey so you made an appointment at the masseuse for Friday after work. After which, by the way, you feel much better, although still sore and tired. Once the evening has passed you fill a tub with hot water, a handful of Epsom salts, and a tea bath soak filled with rosemary. The salts help relax your muscles even more and soften your skin at the same time, the rosemary's aroma is relaxing and the tea it's is helping to circulate your blood increasing healing and relaxation.

With a better understanding of holistic wellness, you are now able to treat your symptoms accordingly. This is not an imagined scenario, you are the leader, the curator, and the boss of your body and you get to choose the right healing methods that work for you.

Chapter checklist

Identify Anti-Inflammatory Herbs that might work for you:

☐ Learn about common anti-inflammatory herbs like turmeric, ginger, and garlic, and understand their benefits and uses.

☐ Explore how to grow these herbs at home and incorporate them into your daily diet.

Understand Anti-Inflammatory Supplements before you take them:

☐ Discover supplements like omega-3 fatty acids, curcumin, and zinc known for their anti-inflammatory properties.

☐ Learn the correct dosages and ways to include them in your routine.

☐ Remember to consult with a healthcare provider before starting any new supplement.

Consider Complementary Therapies:

☐ Explore natural remedies such as acupuncture, massage therapy, hydrotherapy, aromatherapy, cryotherapy, and biofeedback.

☐ Understand how these therapies can reduce inflammation and improve overall health.

How you can connect more with nature:

☐ Delve into the concept of ecotherapy and its benefits for reducing stress and inflammation.

☐ Find simple ways to increase your exposure to nature, such as gardening or visiting local parks.

With a newfound appreciation for nature's pharmacy and its role in reducing inflammation, you're now equipped with a wealth of knowledge about herbs, supplements, and natural therapies. Altogether, you have a better understanding of a holistic path toward taming inflammation for good from diet to movement to mindfulness to using herbs and supplements, you are now armed to take the final step in this journey toward healing.

In the next chapter, we will finally solidify your plan for your journey and focus on putting this knowledge into action. In the next chapter, we guide you through establishing a personalized, practical plan to reduce chronic inflammation. Through a four-week challenge, you'll have the opportunity to apply the insights gained from this book and start walking a sustainable path toward improved health and well-being. Are you ready? Let's go!

Chapter 8 - C.A.L.M.N.E.S.**S.**

S - Solidify an Action Plan

"A healthy lifestyle is the most potent medicine at your disposal."

Dr. Sravani Saha Nakhro

This statement should be much clearer now than it would have been at the beginning of this book. You should now have a clear understanding that health is influenced by genetics, as well as our working and living environments. At the end of the day, you get to choose how to treat and ultimately heal your body. You are the ringmaster of your journey, and I hope you feel equipped and ready to win the fight against inflammation. Now I have a challenge for you. But fear not! You already have a solid understanding of holistic health and wellness. We just need to put that knowledge into action. Knowing is one thing, but doing is how we achieve our goals, create habits, and ultimately begin to heal.

4-week anti-inflammatory challenge

Week 1: Diet and Hydration

Goals:

- Replace processed foods with whole foods.
- Introduce more anti-inflammatory foods (berries, leafy greens, nuts, fatty fish).
- Increase water intake to at least 8 glasses a day.

Daily Actions:

Day 1-7:

o   Add at least one new anti-inflammatory food to your meals each day.
o   Replace one sugary drink with water or herbal tea.
o   Keep a food and hydration diary to track your intake.

Grocery Ideas

Fruits:

- Berries (blueberries, strawberries, raspberries)
- Cherries
- Apples
- Oranges

Vegetables:

- Leafy greens (spinach, kale, Swiss chard)
- Broccoli
- Brussels sprouts
- Sweet potatoes

Proteins:

- Fatty fish (salmon, mackerel, sardines)
- Lean meats (chicken, turkey)
- Legumes (beans, lentils)
- Nuts and seeds (walnuts, almonds, chia seeds)

Grains:

- Whole grains (quinoa, brown rice, oats)
- Whole grain bread
- Whole grain pasta

Dairy and Alternatives:

- Greek yogurt
- Almond milk
- Cottage cheese

Spices and Herbs:

- Turmeric
- Ginger
- Garlic
- Cinnamon

Beverages:

- Green tea
- Herbal tea
- Coconut water

Healthy Fats:

- Olive oil
- Avocados

<u>Sample Meals:</u>

Breakfast:

- Greek yogurt with berries and chia seeds.
- Oatmeal topped with walnuts, sliced apples, and a sprinkle of cinnamon.

Lunch:

- Spinach and kale salad with grilled chicken, cherry tomatoes, and an olive oil vinaigrette.
- Quinoa bowl with roasted sweet potatoes, black beans, avocado, and a turmeric dressing.

Dinner:

- Baked salmon with a side of steamed broccoli and brown

rice.

- Stir-fried vegetables (bell peppers, broccoli, carrots) with tofu and ginger-garlic sauce over whole grain noodles.

Snacks:

- A handful of almonds or walnuts.
- Sliced bell peppers with hummus.
- A piece of fruit (apple, orange).

<u>Tips for Success:</u>

- Meal Prep: Spend some time planning and preparing your meals ahead of time to ensure you have healthy options readily available.

- Hydration: Carry a water bottle with you to stay hydrated throughout the day.

- Mindful Eating: Pay attention to your body's hunger and fullness cues, and try to eat slowly and mindfully.

(2-week meal plan example in the next section of this chapter)

Week 2: Physical Activity

Goals:

- Incorporate at least 30 minutes of moderate exercise into your daily routine.
- Try different types of exercises that encourage flexibility, strength, and endurance.

Daily Actions:

Day 1-7:

o   Schedule a specific time each day for your exercise to establish a routine.
o   Explore one new form of physical activity this week to find what you enjoy.
o   Continue with your dietary improvements and hydration from

Week 1.
Types of Exercises:

Cardiovascular:

- Walking: A brisk 30-minute walk in your neighborhood or at a local park.
- Cycling: A 30-minute bike ride, either outdoors or on a stationary bike.
- Swimming: 30 minutes of swimming or water aerobics.

Strength Training:

- Bodyweight exercises: Squats, lunges, push-ups, and planks.
- Resistance bands: Incorporate resistance band exercises to build muscle.
- Light weights: Use dumbbells for exercises like bicep curls, tricep extensions, and shoulder presses.

Flexibility and Balance:

- Yoga: Follow a beginner's yoga routine for 30 minutes.
- Pilates: Engage in a 30-minute Pilates session focusing on core strength.
- Tai Chi: Practice Tai Chi for relaxation and balance.

Sample Weekly Exercise Plan:

1. Monday: 30-minute brisk walk.
2. Tuesday: 30-minute bodyweight workout (squats, lunges, push-ups, planks).
3. Wednesday: 30-minute yoga session.
4. Thursday: 30-minute cycling session.
5. Friday: 30-minute resistance band workout.
6. Saturday: 30-minute swimming session.
7. Sunday: 30-minute Tai Chi practice.

Tips for Success:

- Consistency: Stick to the same time each day to build a habit.
- Variety: Mix different types of exercises to keep your routine

interesting and work different muscle groups.
- Listen to Your Body: Pay attention to how your body feels and adjust the intensity of your workouts accordingly.
- Progress Tracking: Keep a log of your workouts to monitor your progress and stay motivated.

Healthy Habits Continuation:

- Diet: Maintain your whole foods and anti-inflammatory diet from Week 1.
- Hydration: Continue drinking at least 8 glasses of water daily.
- Rest: Ensure you get enough rest and recovery, especially after intense workouts.

By the end of Week 2, you will have established a regular exercise routine that complements your anti-inflammatory diet and hydration habits from Week 1. This combination will help you build a solid foundation for a healthier lifestyle.

Week 3: Stress Management and Sleep

Goals:

- Practice stress-reduction techniques daily (mindfulness, deep breathing, or meditation).
- Aim for 7-9 hours of quality sleep each night by establishing a consistent sleep schedule.

Daily Actions:

Day 1-7:

o Dedicate 10-15 minutes each day to mindfulness or meditation.
o Turn off electronic devices at least one hour before bedtime.
o Create a relaxing bedtime routine (reading, taking a warm bath).
o Maintain the dietary and physical activity habits established

in Weeks 1 and 2.

Stress-Reduction Techniques:

Mindfulness Meditation

- Basic Practice: Sit comfortably, close your eyes, and focus on your breath. When your mind wanders, gently bring your focus back to your breath.
- Body Scan: Lie down or sit comfortably and slowly bring your attention to each part of your body, starting from your toes and moving up to your head.

Deep Breathing

- 4-7-8 Technique: Inhale through your nose for 4 seconds, hold your breath for 7 seconds, and exhale through your mouth for 8 seconds.
- Belly Breathing: Place one hand on your chest and the other on your belly. Take a deep breath in, allowing your belly to rise, and then exhale slowly.

Progressive Muscle Relaxation

- Tensing and Releasing: Start with your toes and work your way up, tensing each muscle group for 5 seconds and then releasing.

Improving Sleep Quality

Sleep Hygiene Tips:

- Consistent Sleep Schedule: Go to bed and wake up at the same time every day, even on weekends.
- Create a Sleep-Inducing Environment: Make your bedroom dark, quiet, and cool. Consider using blackout curtains and a white noise machine.
- Limit Stimulants: Avoid caffeine and nicotine in the hours leading up to bedtime.
- Evening Routine: Engage in calming activities like reading, taking a warm bath, or listening to soothing music.

Sample Weekly Stress Management and Sleep Plan

Monday:

- 10 minutes of mindfulness meditation.
- Turn off electronics an hour before bed.
- Read a book for 20 minutes before sleeping.

Tuesday:

- Practice deep breathing for 10 minutes.
- Take a warm bath before bed.
- Ensure the bedroom is dark and quiet.

Wednesday:

- Do a body scan meditation for 15 minutes.
- Write in a journal for 20 minutes before sleeping.
- Maintain a consistent sleep schedule.

Thursday:

- Practice the 4-7-8 breathing technique for 10 minutes.
- Avoid caffeine in the evening.
- Listen to soothing music before bed.

Friday:

- Engage in progressive muscle relaxation for 15 minutes.
- Turn off electronics an hour before bed.
- Create a to-do list for the next day to clear your mind.

Saturday:

- Spend 15 minutes in nature, practicing mindfulness.
- Take a warm bath before bed.
- Maintain a consistent sleep schedule.

Sunday:

- Combine body scan and deep breathing for 15 minutes.
- Read a book or write in a journal before sleeping.
- Review your week and reflect on any progress in your stress levels and sleep quality.

Tips for Success:

- Consistency: Practice stress-reduction techniques daily to build a habit.

- Routine: Establish a regular evening routine to signal to your body that it's time to wind down.

- Environment: Create a sleep-friendly environment to enhance the quality of your sleep.

- Progress Tracking: Keep a journal to monitor your stress levels and sleep quality, noting any improvements or challenges.

By the end of Week 3, you will have incorporated effective stress management techniques and established healthy sleep habits, further reducing inflammation and promoting overall well-being. Continue to build on your dietary and physical activity practices from the previous weeks for a holistic approach to health.

Week 4: Lifestyle Adjustments

Goals:

- Reduce or eliminate the consumption of alcohol and tobacco.
- Incorporate daily self-care activities that promote relaxation and joy.
- Review and adjust your goals based on what you've learned about your body's responses over the past weeks.

Daily Actions:

Day 1-7:

- Choose a self-care activity to practice daily (hobbies, spending time in nature, etc.).
- If you consume alcohol or tobacco, reduce the amount gradually and note any changes in how you feel.
- Reflect on your progress and any changes in symptoms of inflammation you've noticed.
- Continue with the dietary, physical activity, and stress management practices from the previous weeks.

Reducing Alcohol and Tobacco:

Alcohol Reduction Tips

- Set Limits: Decide how many days a week you will drink and set a limit on the number of drinks.
- Alternatives: Replace alcoholic drinks with non-alcoholic options like sparkling water, herbal tea, or mocktails.
- Mindfulness: Pay attention to the reasons why you drink and find healthier alternatives to cope with stress or social situations.

Tobacco Reduction Tips:

- Gradual Reduction: Cut down the number of cigarettes you smoke each day or use nicotine replacement therapy.
- Support Systems: Seek support from friends, family, or support groups.
- Stress Management: Replace smoking with stress-reduction techniques learned in Week 3, such as deep breathing or mindfulness.

Incorporating Daily Self-Care Activities:

Self-Care Activities:

- Hobbies: Engage in activities you enjoy, such as reading, painting, gardening, or playing a musical instrument.
- Nature: Spend time in nature, whether it's a walk in the park, hiking, or simply sitting in your garden.
- Social Connections: Spend quality time with family and friends to strengthen social bonds and reduce stress.
- Relaxation: Practice relaxation techniques such as yoga, tai chi, or taking a warm bath.

Sample Weekly Lifestyle Adjustment Plan:

Monday:

- Choose a new self-care activity to try, such as painting or journaling.
- Reduce alcohol intake by replacing evening drinks with herbal tea.
- Reflect on your progress in a journal.

Tuesday:

- Spend 30 minutes in nature, whether it's a walk in the park or

gardening.
- Reduce tobacco consumption by smoking one less cigarette.
- Continue practicing mindfulness meditation.

Wednesday:

- Engage in a hobby you enjoy for 30 minutes.
- Replace another alcoholic drink with a non-alcoholic alternative.
- Review your food and hydration diary from Week 1.

Thursday:

- Practice yoga or tai chi for relaxation.
- Further reduce tobacco consumption by replacing smoking with deep breathing exercises.
- Turn off electronics an hour before bed and practice your sleep routine.

Friday:

- Spend quality time with family or friends.
- Reflect on any changes in inflammation symptoms and overall well-being.
- Continue with dietary improvements and physical activity.

Saturday:

- Try a new self-care activity, such as cooking a healthy meal or visiting a new place.
- Continue to monitor and reduce alcohol and tobacco intake.
- Engage in a body scan meditation before bed.

Sunday:

- Review your progress over the past four weeks.
- Set new goals based on what you have learned about your body's responses.
- Continue with all the healthy habits established throughout the challenge.

Tips for Success:

- Consistency: Consistently practice self-care activities and reduce alcohol and tobacco consumption.

- Support: Seek support from friends, family, or support groups to stay motivated.

- Reflection: Regularly reflect on your progress and adjust your goals as needed.

- Holistic Approach: Maintain the dietary, physical activity, and stress management practices from previous weeks for a comprehensive approach to reducing inflammation.

By the end of Week 4, you will have made significant lifestyle adjustments that promote relaxation and joy, further contributing to reducing inflammation. Reflect on your journey, celebrate your successes, and continue building on these habits for long-term health and well-being.

Week 1

Day 1:

- Breakfast: Smoothie with spinach, mango, almond milk, and chia seeds
- Lunch: Mixed green salad with grilled chicken, avocado, cherry tomatoes, and lemon vinaigrette
- Dinner: Baked cod with roasted carrots and quinoa

Day 2:

- Breakfast: Overnight oats with almond milk, flaxseeds, and blueberries
- Lunch: Lentil and vegetable soup with a side of whole-grain bread
- Dinner: Grilled tofu with sautéed kale and brown rice

Day 3:

- Breakfast: Greek yogurt parfait with granola, strawberries, and a drizzle of honey
- Lunch: Turkey and avocado wrap with whole-grain tortilla
- Dinner: Shrimp stir-fry with mixed vegetables and soba noodles

Day 4:

- Breakfast: Chia pudding with coconut milk and raspberries
- Lunch: Quinoa salad with cucumbers, tomatoes, olives, and feta cheese
- Dinner: Grilled salmon with steamed asparagus and sweet potato mash

Day 5:

- Breakfast: Smoothie bowl with mixed berries, almond butter, and granola
- Lunch: Chickpea and vegetable curry with brown rice
- Dinner: Baked chicken thighs with roasted Brussels sprouts and wild rice

Day 6:

- Breakfast: Whole-grain toast with avocado and a poached egg
- Lunch: Spinach and feta stuffed portobello mushrooms
- Dinner: Baked trout with garlic green beans and quinoa

Day 7:

- Breakfast: Oatmeal with almonds, banana slices, and a drizzle of maple syrup
- Lunch: Roasted vegetable and hummus wrap with whole-grain tortilla
- Dinner: Beef and broccoli stir-fry with brown rice

Week 2

Day 8:

- Breakfast: Smoothie with kale, pineapple, coconut water, and chia seeds
- Lunch: Tomato basil soup with a side salad
- Dinner: Grilled shrimp with quinoa and sautéed spinach

Day 9:

- Breakfast: Greek yogurt with granola, honey, and fresh berries
- Lunch: Quinoa with mixed fresh herbs, cucumbers, and tomatoes
- Dinner: Baked chicken breast with roasted sweet potatoes and green beans

Day 10:

- Breakfast: Chia seed pudding with almond milk and mango
- Lunch: Lentil and vegetable stew
- Dinner: Baked salmon with steamed broccoli and wild rice

Day 11:

- Breakfast: Whole-grain toast with almond butter and sliced banana

- Lunch: Mediterranean chickpea salad with feta cheese and olives
- Dinner: Grilled tofu with stir-fried vegetables and brown rice

Day 12:

- Breakfast: Smoothie bowl with spinach, berries, and flaxseeds
- Lunch: Spinach and mushroom omelet with a side of whole-grain toast
- Dinner: Baked trout with roasted root vegetables and quinoa

Day 13:

- Breakfast: Overnight oats with almond milk, chia seeds, and blueberries
- Lunch: Roasted vegetable and chickpea bowl
- Dinner: Grilled chicken thighs with roasted butternut squash and asparagus

Day 14:

- Breakfast: Greek yogurt parfait with granola and mixed berries
- Lunch: Hummus and veggie wrap with whole-grain tortilla
- Dinner: Zucchini noodles with pesto sauce and cherry tomatoes

Grocery List:

Proteins:

- Salmon
- Chicken breast
- Tofu
- Shrimp
- Greek yogurt
- Eggs
- Lentils
- Chickpeas
- Ground turkey
- Cod

- Trout
- Beef (for stir-fry)

Vegetables:

- Spinach
- Kale
- Broccoli
- Sweet potatoes
- Bell peppers
- Brussels sprouts
- Mixed greens
- Avocado
- Tomatoes
- Cucumbers
- Mushrooms
- Zucchini
- Asparagus
- Carrots
- Green beans

Fruits:

- Berries (strawberries, blueberries, raspberries)
- Bananas
- Apples
- Mango
- Pineapple
- Lemon

Grains and Legumes:

- Quinoa
- Brown rice
- Whole-grain bread
- Whole-grain tortillas
- Soba noodles
- Wild rice
- Oats
- Black beans
- Chickpeas

Nuts and Seeds:

- Walnuts
- Chia seeds
- Flaxseeds
- Almonds
- Almond butter

Others:

- Olive oil
- Herbal teas
- Almond milk
- Coconut milk
- Hummus
- Feta cheese
- Pesto
- Granola

This plan provides a wide variety of nutrient-dense, anti-inflammatory foods, ensuring meals are balanced and enjoyable.

Anti-inflammatory Recipes to try

In combination with the meal plans already provided, use these recipes to create meal plans to continue your healthy journey toward an anti-inflammatory lifestyle.

5 Anti-Inflammatory Recipes for Breakfast

1.Spinach and Feta Scrambled Egg Pitas

Ingredients:

- 2 large eggs
- 1/2 cup fresh spinach, chopped
- 1/4 cup crumbled feta cheese
- 1 whole-grain pita, cut in half
- Salt and pepper, to taste
- 1 tsp olive oil

Instructions:

1. Heat olive oil in a non-stick skillet over medium heat.
2. Add chopped spinach and sauté until wilted.
3. In a bowl, whisk eggs with salt and pepper.
4. Pour eggs into the skillet and scramble until cooked through.
5. Stir in feta cheese.
6. Stuff the scrambled eggs into pita halves and serve warm.

2. Blueberry Avocado Smoothie

Ingredients:

- 1/2 avocado
- 1 cup frozen blueberries
- 1 cup unsweetened almond milk
- 1 tbsp chia seeds
- 1 tbsp honey (optional)

Instructions:

1. Place all ingredients in a blender.
2. Blend until smooth and creamy.
3. Pour into a glass and enjoy immediately.

3. Smoked Trout and Spinach Egg Scramble

Ingredients:

- 2 large eggs
- 1/2 cup fresh spinach, chopped
- 1/4 cup smoked trout, flaked
- Salt and pepper, to taste
- 1 tsp olive oil

Instructions:

1. Heat olive oil in a non-stick skillet over medium heat.
2. Add chopped spinach and sauté until wilted.
3. In a bowl, whisk eggs with salt and pepper.
4. Pour eggs into the skillet and scramble until almost set.

5. Add flaked smoked trout and continue to cook until eggs are fully set.
6. Serve warm.

4.Mango Almond Smoothie Bowl

Ingredients:

- 1 cup frozen mango chunks
- 1/2 cup unsweetened almond milk
- 1/4 cup Greek yogurt
- 1 tbsp almond butter
- 1 tsp honey (optional)
- Toppings: sliced almonds, chia seeds, fresh berries

Instructions:

1. Blend mango, almond milk, Greek yogurt, almond butter, and honey until smooth.
2. Pour the mixture into a bowl.
3. Top with sliced almonds, chia seeds, and fresh berries.
4. Serve immediately.

5. Breakfast Beans with Microwave Poached Egg

Ingredients:

- 1/2 cup canned black beans, rinsed and drained
- 1/2 cup diced tomatoes
- 1/4 tsp cumin
- 1/4 tsp paprika
- Salt and pepper, to taste
- 1 large egg
- 1 tsp vinegar
- Fresh cilantro, for garnish

Instructions:

1. In a microwave-safe bowl, mix black beans, diced tomatoes, cumin, paprika, salt, and pepper.
2. Microwave on high for 2 minutes, stirring halfway through.
3. Fill a microwave-safe mug with 1/2 cup water and add

vinegar.

4. Crack the egg into the mug and microwave on high for 1 minute.

5. Drain the egg and place it on top of the beans.

6. Garnish with fresh cilantro and serve.

5 Anti-Inflammatory Recipes for Lunch

1. Chicken Avocado Ranch Naan

Ingredients:

- 1 whole-grain naan
- 1/2 avocado, sliced
- 1/2 cup cooked chicken breast, shredded
- 2 tbsp ranch dressing
- 1/4 cup cherry tomatoes, halved
- Fresh cilantro, for garnish

Instructions:

1. Preheat the oven to 375°F (190°C).
2. Place the naan on a baking sheet.
3. Spread ranch dressing evenly over the naan.
4. Top with shredded chicken, avocado slices, and cherry tomatoes.
5. Bake for 10 minutes or until the naan is crispy.
6. Garnish with fresh cilantro and serve warm.

2. Instant Pot Lentils

Ingredients:

- 1 cup dried lentils, rinsed
- 3 cups vegetable broth
- 1 onion, diced
- 2 cloves garlic, minced
- 1 tsp cumin
- 1 tsp turmeric
- Salt and pepper, to taste

Instructions:

1. Add all ingredients to the Instant Pot.
2. Close the lid and set the pressure release valve to sealing.
3. Cook on high pressure for 15 minutes.
4. Let the pressure release naturally for 10 minutes, then quickly release any remaining pressure.
5. Stir well and serve.

3. Best Tuna Salad Sandwich

Ingredients:

- 1 can tuna, drained
- 2 tbsp Greek yogurt
- 1 tbsp Dijon mustard
- 1 celery stalk, diced
- 1/4 red onion, diced
- Salt and pepper, to taste
- 2 slices whole-grain bread
- Lettuce leaves

Instructions:

1. In a bowl, mix tuna, Greek yogurt, dijon mustard, celery, red onion, salt, and pepper.
2. Spread the tuna salad evenly on one slice of whole-grain bread.
3. Top with lettuce leaves and the other slice of bread.
4. Cut in half and serve.

4. Cucumber Roasted Red Pepper Wrap

Ingredients:

- 1 whole-grain tortilla
- 1/2 cucumber, sliced
- 1/4 cup roasted red peppers, sliced
- 2 tbsp hummus
- 1/4 cup baby spinach leaves
- Salt and pepper, to taste

Instructions:

1. Lay the tortilla flat and spread hummus evenly over it.
2. Arrange cucumber slices, roasted red peppers, and spinach leaves on top.
3. Season with salt and pepper.
4. Roll up the tortilla tightly and slice in half.
5. Serve immediately.

5. Lemonade Shrimp Kale and Potato Salad

Ingredients:

- 1 cup shrimp, cooked and peeled
- 2 cups kale, chopped
- 1 cup baby potatoes, boiled and halved
- 1/4 cup red onion, thinly sliced
- 1 lemon, juiced
- 2 tbsp olive oil
- Salt and pepper, to taste

Instructions:

1. In a large bowl, combine shrimp, kale, baby potatoes, and red onion.
2. In a small bowl, whisk together lemon juice, olive oil, salt, and pepper.
3. Pour the dressing over the salad and toss to coat evenly.
4. Serve chilled or at room temperature.

5 Anti-Inflammatory Recipes for Supper

1. Spicy Chicken and Sweet Potato Stew

Ingredients:

- 1 lb chicken breast, cut into chunks
- 2 sweet potatoes, peeled and cubed
- 1 onion, diced
- 2 cloves garlic, minced
- 1 red bell pepper, diced
- 1 can diced tomatoes

- 2 cups chicken broth
- 1 tsp cumin
- 1 tsp smoked paprika
- 1/2 tsp cayenne pepper
- Salt and pepper, to taste
- 2 tbsp olive oil
- Fresh cilantro, for garnish

Instructions:

1. Heat olive oil in a large pot over medium heat. Add chicken and cook until browned.
2. Add onion, garlic, and red bell pepper. Cook until softened.
3. Stir in sweet potatoes, diced tomatoes, chicken broth, cumin, smoked paprika, cayenne pepper, salt, and pepper.
4. Bring to a boil, then reduce heat and simmer for 20-25 minutes until sweet potatoes are tender.
5. Garnish with fresh cilantro and serve.

2. Salmon with Ginger Glaze

Ingredients:

- 4 salmon filets
- 2 tbsp soy sauce
- 2 tbsp honey
- 1 tbsp grated ginger
- 2 cloves garlic, minced
- 1 tbsp rice vinegar
- 1 tsp sesame oil
- 1 tbsp olive oil
- Sesame seeds and green onions, for garnish

Instructions:

1. In a bowl, mix soy sauce, honey, ginger, garlic, rice vinegar, and sesame oil.
2. Heat olive oil in a skillet over medium heat.
3. Add salmon filets, skin-side down, and cook for 4-5 minutes.
4. Flip salmon and pour the glaze over the filets.
5. Cook for an additional 4-5 minutes until the salmon is cooked through and the glaze is thickened.

6. Garnish with sesame seeds and green onions before serving.

3. Grilled Cauliflower Steaks

Ingredients:

- 1 large cauliflower head, sliced into 1-inch thick steaks
- 3 tbsp olive oil
- 1 tsp smoked paprika
- 1 tsp garlic powder
- Salt and pepper, to taste
- Fresh parsley, for garnish

Instructions:

1. Preheat the grill to medium-high heat.
2. In a bowl, mix olive oil, smoked paprika, garlic powder, salt, and pepper.
3. Brush cauliflower steaks with the olive oil mixture.
4. Grill cauliflower steaks for 5-7 minutes on each side until tender and slightly charred.
5. Garnish with fresh parsley and serve.

4. Quinoa Vegetable Soup

Ingredients:

- 1 cup quinoa, rinsed
- 1 onion, diced
- 2 cloves garlic, minced
- 3 carrots, sliced
- 2 celery stalks, sliced
- 1 zucchini, diced
- 1 can diced tomatoes
- 4 cups vegetable broth
- 1 tsp dried thyme
- 1 tsp dried oregano
- Salt and pepper, to taste
- 2 tbsp olive oil
- Fresh parsley, for garnish

Instructions:

1. Heat olive oil in a large pot over medium heat. Add onion and garlic, cooking until softened.
2. Add carrots, celery, and zucchini, and cook for 5 minutes.
3. Stir in quinoa, diced tomatoes, vegetable broth, thyme, oregano, salt, and pepper.
4. Bring to a boil, then reduce heat and simmer for 20-25 minutes until vegetables and quinoa are tender.
5. Garnish with fresh parsley and serve.

5. Butternut Squash with Ginger and Quinoa

Ingredients:

- 1 butternut squash, peeled and cubed
- 1 cup quinoa, rinsed
- 1 onion, diced
- 2 cloves garlic, minced
- 1 tbsp grated ginger
- 2 cups vegetable broth
- 2 tbsp olive oil
- Salt and pepper, to taste
- Fresh cilantro, for garnish

Instructions:

1. Preheat the oven to 400°F (200°C). Toss butternut squash with 1 tbsp olive oil, salt, and pepper. Roast for 25-30 minutes until tender.
2. In a pot, heat remaining olive oil over medium heat. Add onion, garlic, and ginger, cooking until softened.
3. Stir in quinoa and vegetable broth. Bring to a boil, then reduce heat and simmer for 15 minutes until quinoa is cooked.
4. Combine roasted butternut squash with quinoa mixture.
5. Garnish with fresh cilantro and serve.

Anti-inflammatory snacks and dessert ideas

Snacks

- Dark chocolate and mixed nuts
- Hummus and raw veggies

- Guacamole and corn chips
- Frozen yogurt bars
- Crispy spiced chickpeas

Desserts

- Apple tart with walnut crust
- Mixed Berries with oat crumble
- Honey (sweet) cornbread with vanilla and coconut ice cream
- Lemon bars with coconut crust
- Fruit parfait with coconut cream sprinkles with granola or toasted coconut shreds

Don't limit yourself because you're on a healing journey. Balance is key, and having a healthy yet delicious treat once in a while is a nice reward for all the good you're doing for your body. Just remember if these foods trigger pain, avoid them, otherwise enjoy life and have a treat once in a while. Try some of the recipes provided and see how Delicious eating healthy can actually be.

Conclusion

In this book we've journeyed through the intricate world of chronic inflammation, arming you with practical strategies to reclaim your health. We started by understanding inflammation's dual nature: its role as both a healer and a potential disruptor when chronic. Recognizing its signs and causes is crucial in this battle.

We then ventured into the kitchen, exploring the power of anti-inflammatory foods like berries, leafy greens, nuts, and fatty fish, coupled with the benefits of proper hydration. Our 4-week challenge guided you to replace processed foods, increase water intake, and incorporate these foods into daily meals.

Exercise became our next focus, revealing how physical activity can reduce inflammation. From yoga and walking to strength training, we highlighted various exercises and provided tips to integrate them into your routine. The fitness assessment helped gauge your fitness level and offered practical solutions to overcome common exercise barriers.

Stress management and sleep emerged as vital components. Chronic stress exacerbates inflammation, so we introduced mindfulness, meditation, and relaxation techniques. Quality sleep's importance was emphasized, with tips to improve sleep hygiene and a look at how sleep affects the immune system.

Lifestyle adjustments, including reducing alcohol and tobacco consumption, were discussed with guidance on moderation and alternatives. Self-care practices were highlighted, with ideas for integrating them into daily routines and fostering a positive mindset.

We explored nature's offerings, from anti-inflammatory herbs like turmeric and ginger to supplements such as omega-3 fatty acids and curcumin. Complementary therapies like acupuncture, massage, hydrotherapy, and aromatherapy were discussed, each playing a role in reducing inflammation and promoting well-being.

Connecting with nature was another key theme. We explored ecotherapy's concept and benefits, suggesting ways to increase nature exposure to enhance mental and physical health.

Finally, our 4-week anti-inflammatory challenge brought everything together, guiding you through dietary changes, exercise, stress reduction, and sleep improvements. Each week focused on a different aspect, with specific tasks and goals to ensure a manageable and sustainable approach to better health.

Throughout this journey, we've likened your immune system to a team of superhero firefighters, tirelessly working to keep inflammation at bay. You're in charge of their environment, and by creating a supportive habitat, you help these heroes perform at their best.

Imagine your immune system as a bustling firehouse. Each white blood cell is a dedicated firefighter, ready to leap into action at the first sign of trouble. Your diet, exercise, and lifestyle choices are the firehouse's maintenance plan, ensuring everything runs smoothly. By choosing anti-inflammatory foods, you're fueling the fire trucks with premium gasoline. Regular exercise keeps the hoses in top shape, ready to douse any flare-ups. Managing stress and getting quality sleep ensure the firefighters are well-rested and alert, prepared for any emergency.

As you move forward, remember that you're the fire chief of your body's firehouse. Keep your team well-supported, and they'll continue to protect you from the flames of inflammation. Embrace the strategies you've learned, stay committed to your health, and enjoy the benefits of a life free from chronic pain, with inflammation under control.

Congratulations on completing this journey! You've armed yourself with the tools you need to tame inflammation and enhance your well-being. Now you can continue supporting your superhero firefighters so your life can be filled with greater vitality and long-lasting health.

Thanks for Reading,
Please Leave a Review!

I would be *incredibly appreciative* if you could rate my book or leave a review on **Amazon**.

Just scan this QR code with your phone, or visit the www.ipreview.smartmindpublishing.com link to land directly on the book's Amazon review page.

Your review not only helps me create better books but also helps more readers succeed in calming their inflammation.

Thank you!

Tara

Bibliography

Chapter 1: Understanding Inflammation

1. National Institute of Arthritis and Musculoskeletal and Skin Diseases. (2020). "What Is Inflammation?" NIAMS.nih.gov.
2. Medzhitov, R. (2008). "Origin and physiological roles of inflammation." Nature, 454(7203), 428-435.
3. Calder, P. C. (2021). "Nutrition, immunity and COVID-19." BMJ Nutrition, Prevention & Health, 3(1), 74-92.

Identifying Chronic Inflammation

1. Hotamisligil, G. S. (2006). "Inflammation and metabolic disorders." Nature, 444(7121), 860-867.
2. Furman, D., Campisi, J., Verdin, E., et al. (2019). "Chronic inflammation in the etiology of disease across the lifespan." Nature Medicine, 25(12), 1822-1832.
3. Libby, P. (2002). "Inflammation in atherosclerosis." Nature, 420(6917), 868-874.
4. Nathan, C., & Ding, A. (2010). "Nonresolving inflammation." Cell, 140(6), 871-882.
5. Furman, D., Chang, J., Lartigue, L., et al. (2017). "Expression of specific inflammasome gene modules stratifies older individuals into two extreme clinical and immunological states." Nature Medicine, 23(2), 174-184.
6. Slavin, J. L. (2005). "Dietary fiber and body weight." Nutrition, 21(3), 411-418.
7. Mrazek, F., Simková, A., & Houska, M. (2017). "Microbial Biofilms and Biofilm Infections in Healthcare." Journal of Microbiology and Infectious Diseases, 7(2), 59-63.

Chapter 2: Anti-inflammatory Diet and Nutrition

1. Calder, P. C. (2013). "Omega-3 polyunsaturated fatty acids and inflammatory processes: Nutrition or pharmacology?" British Journal of Clinical Pharmacology, 75(3), 645-662.
2. Holt, E. M., Steffen, L. M., Moran, A., et al. (2009). "Fruit

and vegetable consumption and its relation to markers of inflammation and oxidative stress in adolescents." Journal of the American Dietetic Association, 109(3), 414-421.

3. Kris-Etherton, P. M., Harris, W. S., & Appel, L. J. (2003). "Fish consumption, fish oil, omega-3 fatty acids, and cardiovascular disease." Circulation, 106(21), 2747-2757.

4. Heber, D. (2014). "Vegetables, fruits and phytoestrogens in the prevention of diseases." Journal of Postgraduate Medicine, 60(3), 260-265.

5. Willett, W. C. (2006). "The Mediterranean diet: Science and practice." Public Health Nutrition, 9(1a), 105-110.

Chapter 3: Leveraging Movement

1. Booth, F. W., Roberts, C. K., & Laye, M. J. (2012). "Lack of exercise is a major cause of chronic diseases." Comprehensive Physiology, 2(2), 1143-1211.

2. Mora, S., Cook, N., Buring, J. E., et al. (2007). "Physical activity and reduced risk of cardiovascular events: potential mediating mechanisms." Circulation, 116(19), 2110-2118.

3. Penedo, F. J., & Dahn, J. R. (2005). "Exercise and well-being: a review of mental and physical health benefits associated with physical activity." Current Opinion in Psychiatry, 18(2), 189-193.

4. Ridker, P. M. (2003). "C-reactive protein: Eighty years from discovery to emergence as a major risk marker for cardiovascular disease." Clinical Chemistry, 49(5), 682-685.

5. Smith, P. J., Blumenthal, J. A., Babyak, M. A., et al. (2010). "Effects of exercise and weight loss on depressive symptoms among men and women with major depression." Journal of Psychosomatic Research, 69(4), 313-318.

Chapter 4: Managing Stress and Emotional Health

1. Steptoe, A., & Kivimäki, M. (2012). "Stress and cardiovascular disease." Nature Reviews Cardiology, 9(6), 360-370.

2. Schneiderman, N., Ironson, G., & Siegel, S. D. (2005). "Stress and health: Psychological, behavioral, and biological determinants." Annual Review of Clinical Psychology, 1, 607-628.

3. Chida, Y., & Steptoe, A. (2009). "The association of anger

and hostility with future coronary heart disease: a meta-analytic review of prospective evidence." Journal of the American College of Cardiology, 53(11), 936-946.

4. Cohen, S., Janicki-Deverts, D., & Miller, G. E. (2007). "Psychological stress and disease." JAMA, 298(14), 1685-1687.

5. McEwen, B. S. (1998). "Protective and damaging effects of stress mediators." New England Journal of Medicine, 338(3), 171-179.

Chapter 5: Inflammation and Sleep

1. Irwin, M. R. (2015). "Why sleep is important for health: a psychoneuroimmunology perspective." Annual Review of Psychology, 66, 143-172.

2. Besedovsky, L., Lange, T., & Born, J. (2012). "Sleep and immune function." Pflugers Archiv-European Journal of Physiology, 463(1), 121-137.

3. Prather, A. A., Janicki-Deverts, D., Hall, M. H., & Cohen, S. (2015). "Behaviorally assessed sleep and susceptibility to the common cold." Sleep, 38(9), 1353-1359.

4. Grandner, M. A., Patel, N. P., Gehrman, P. R., et al. (2010). "Who gets the best sleep? Ethnic and socioeconomic factors related to sleep complaints." Sleep Medicine, 11(5), 470-478.

5. Irwin, M. R., Olmstead, R., & Carroll, J. E. (2016). "Sleep disturbance, sleep duration, and inflammation: A systematic review and meta-analysis of cohort studies and experimental sleep deprivation." Biological Psychiatry, 80(1), 40-52.

6. Hunter, D. J., & Felson, D. T. (2006). "Osteoarthritis." BMJ, 332(7542), 639-642.

7. Davignon, J., & Ganz, P. (2004). "Role of endothelial dysfunction in atherosclerosis." Circulation, 109(23_suppl_1), III-27.

Chapter 6: Enhanced lifestyle choices

1. Vickers, A., & Zollman, C. (1999). "Herbal medicine." BMJ, 319(7216), 1050-1053.

2. Barnes, P. M., Powell-Griner, E., McFann, K., & Nahin, R. L. (2004). "Complementary and alternative medicine use among adults: United States, 2002." Seminars in Integrative Medicine, 2(2), 54-71.

3. Ernst, E. (2000). "The role of complementary and alternative

medicine." BMJ, 321(7269), 1133-1135.
4. Fønnebø, V., Grimsgaard, S., Walach, H., et al. (2007). "Researching complementary and alternative treatments–the gatekeepers are not at home." BMC Medical Research Methodology, 7(1), 7.
5. Berman, B. M., Langevin, H. M., Witt, C. M., & Dubner, R. (2010). "Acupuncture for chronic low back pain." New England Journal of Medicine, 363(5), 454-461.

Chapter 7: Natural remedies and Nature's pharmacy

1. Indoor Air Quality (IAQ). (2021). "Improving Indoor Air Quality." Environmental Protection Agency (EPA). EPA.gov.
2. Kuo, F. E., & Taylor, A. F. (2004). "A potential natural treatment for Attention-Deficit/Hyperactivity Disorder: Evidence from a national study." American Journal of Public Health, 94(9), 1580-1586.
3. Kaplan, R. (2001). "The nature of the view from home: Psychological benefits." Environment and Behavior, 33(4), 507-542.
4. Sacks, O. (2007). "Musicophilia: Tales of Music and the Brain." Random House.
5. Beatley, T. (2011). "Biophilic Cities: Integrating Nature into Urban Design and Planning." Island Press.

Natural Remedies and Supplements

1. Ernst, E. (2006). "Herbal medicines: balancing benefits and risks." Advances in Pharmacological Sciences, 2006, 929310.
2. Linde, K., Ramirez, G., Mulrow, C. D., et al. (1996). "St John's wort for depression—an overview and meta-analysis of randomised clinical trials." BMJ, 313(7052), 253-258.
3. Valli, G., & Giardina, E. G. V. (2002). "Benefits, adverse effects, and drug interactions of herbal therapies with cardiovascular effects." Journal of the American College of Cardiology, 39(7), 1083-1095.
4. Posadzki, P., Watson, L., & Ernst, E. (2013). "Herbal medicines for the treatment of rheumatoid arthritis: a systematic review of randomized controlled trials." Rheumatology International, 33(1), 111-124.
5. Cochrane Library. (2020). "Cochrane Reviews on Supplements." Cochrane.org.

Chapter 8: Practical Steps for Long-Term Inflammation Management

1. Centers for Disease Control and Prevention (CDC). (2020). "Physical Activity Basics." CDC.gov. CDC.gov.
2. Harvard Health Publishing. (2018). "The importance of staying hydrated." Harvard Health Blog. Harvard.edu.
3. Mayo Clinic Staff. (2019). "Chronic stress puts your health at risk." Mayo Clinic. MayoClinic.org.
4. MedlinePlus. (2020). "Healthy Eating." MedlinePlus. MedlinePlus.gov.
5. National Sleep Foundation. (2019). "How Much Sleep Do We Really Need?" Sleep Foundation. SleepFoundation.org.

Recipes for Anti-Inflammatory Living

1. EatingWell. (2023). "Three-Step Anti-Inflammatory Lunch Recipes." EatingWell. EatingWell.com.
2. Clean Plates. (2023). "Anti-Inflammatory Lunch Recipes." Clean Plates. CleanPlates.com.
3. Allrecipes. (2023). "Anti-Inflammatory Dinner Recipes." Allrecipes. Allrecipes.com.
4. EatingWell. (2023). "Anti-Inflammatory Dinner Recipes in 30 Minutes." EatingWell. EatingWell.com.
5. Mayo Clinic. (2020). "Anti-inflammatory diet: What to know." Mayo Clinic. MayoClinic.org.

Made in the USA
Monee, IL
25 October 2024

68650921R10090